THE TRUTH ABOUT RAPE

SECOND EDITION

Robert N. Golden, M.D.
University of Wisconsin–Madison
General Editor

Fred L. Peterson, Ph.D.
University of Texas–Austin
General Editor

Kathryn Hilgenkamp
Contributing Author

Judith Harper
Contributing Author

Elizabeth Boskey
Contributing Author

William Kane, Ph.D.
University of New Mexico
Adviser to the First Edition

Mark J. Kittleson, Ph.D.
Southern Illinois University
Adviser to the First Edition

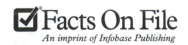
Facts On File
An imprint of Infobase Publishing

The Truth About Rape, Second Edition

Facts On File, Inc.
An imprint of Infobase Publishing
132 West 31st Street
New York, NY 10001

Library of Congress Cataloging-in-Publication Data

The truth about rape / Robert N. Golden, general editor, Fred Peterson, general editor; Kathryn Hilgenkamp, contributing author . . . [et al.]. – 2nd ed.
    p. cm.
  First ed. of this work was edited by Mark J. Kittleson.
  Includes index.
  ISBN-13: 978-0-8160-7642-0 (hardcover : alk. paper)
  ISBN-10: 0-8160-7642-1 (hardcover : alk. paper) 1. Rape. 2. Rape–United States.
I. Golden, Robert N. II. Peterson, Fred. III. Hilgenkamp, Kathryn, 1952–
  HV6558.T73 2010
  362.883–dc22

                                    2009018452

Facts On File books are available at special discounts when purchased in bulk quantities for businesses, associations, institutions, or sales promotions. Please call our Special Sales Department in New York at (212) 967-8800 or (800) 322-8755.

You can find Facts On File on the World Wide Web at
http://www.factsonfile.com.

Text design by David Strelecky
Composition by Mary Susan Ryan-Flynn
Cover printed by Art Print, Taylor, PA
Book printed and bound by Maple Press, York, PA
Date printed: February 2010
Printed in the United States of America

10 9 8 7 6 5 4 3 2 1

This book is printed on acid-free paper and contains 30 percent postconsumer recycled content.

CONTENTS

List of Illustrations and Tables   v

Preface   vii

How to Use This Book   xi

Society and Victims of Rape   1

A–to–Z Entries   **13**

  Abusive Sexual Behavior   15

  Children and Rape   19

  Date Rape   25

  Drugs, Alcohol, and Rape   36

  Educating the Community   41

  Female Rights   46

  Gang Rape   53

  Help and Support   58

  Internet Predators   64

  Law and Rape, The   71

  Male Role in Rape   75

  Prevention of Rape: Being Proactive   83

  Prevention of Rape: Being Reactive   91

  Rape and Religion   96

Rape and Society   99
Rape in the Media, Reporting   105
Rape in War   108
Rape Kits and Evidence Collection   111
Rape Statistics   116
Rape Within Abusive Relationships   123
Safe Areas, Establishing   129
Sexual Abuse in Institutions   134
Sexual Assault, Types of   139
Sexual Harassment   146
Sexual Violence and Children   151
Statutory Rape   154
Stigma of Rape   160
Victims of Rape: Female   165
Victims of Rape: Male   168

Hotlines and Help Sites   173
Glossary   177
Index   183

LIST OF ILLUSTRATIONS AND TABLES

Correlation Between Those Abused as Juveniles
and Future Crime   17

Juvenile Victims of Sexual Abuse   20

The Sexual Victimization of College Women   26

Alcohol Use by Those Convicted of Rape
and Sexual Assault   35

The Most Underreported Violent Crime in America   40

Sex of Victims and Perpetrators of Rape   60

Sexual Solicitation on the Internet of Adolescents,
Aged 10–17   65

Risk Factors for Sexual Violence   76

Rape Rates in the United States   85

New Mexico Sexual Assault Nurse Examiner Program
Helps Law Enforcement   115

Injury During Rape   118

Attacker's Relationship to Victim   124

Sexual Violence in Juvenile Facilities   135

History of Abuse Before Admission to Prison   137

Types of Sexual Crimes 143

State Laws Governing Statutory Rape v.
the Legal Age of Consent 156

Legal Age of Consent in the United States 157

Underreported Crimes: Sexual Abuse 166

Age of First Sexual Assault 167

PREFACE

THE TRUTH ABOUT series—updated and expanded to include 20 volumes—seeks to identify the most pressing health issues and social challenges confronting our nation's youth. Adolescence is the period between the onset of puberty and the attainment of adult roles and responsibilities. Adolescence is also a time of storm, stress, and risk-taking for many young people. During adolescence, a person's health is influenced by biological, psychological, and social factors, all of which interact with one's environment—family, peers, school, and community. It is a time when teenagers experience profound changes.

With the latest available statistics and new insights that have emerged from ongoing research, the Truth About series seeks to help young people build a foundation of information as they face some of the challenges that will affect their health and well-being. These challenges include high-risk behaviors, such as alcohol, tobacco, and other drug use; sexual behaviors that can lead to adolescent pregnancy and sexually transmitted diseases (STDs), such as HIV/AIDS; mental health concerns, such as depression and suicide; learning disorders and disabilities, which are often associated with school failures and school drop-outs; serious family problems, including domestic violence and abuse; and lifestyle factors, which increase adolescents' risk for noncommunicable diseases, such as diabetes and cardiovascular disease, among others.

Broader underlying factors also influence adolescent health. These include socioeconomic circumstances, such as poverty, available health care, and the political and social situations in which young people live. Although these factors can negatively affect adolescent health and well-being, as well as school performance, many of these negative health outcomes are preventable with the proper knowledge and information.

With prevention in mind, the writers and editors of each topical volume in the Truth About series have tried to provide cutting-edge information that is supported by research and scientific evidence. Vital facts are presented that inform youth about the challenges experienced during adolescence, while special features seek to dispel common myths and misconceptions. Some of the main topics explored include abuse, alcohol, death and dying, divorce, drugs, eating disorders, family life, fear and depression, rape, sexual behavior and unplanned pregnancy, smoking, and violence. All volumes discuss risk-taking behaviors and their consequences, healthy choices, prevention, available treatments, and where to get help.

In this new edition of the series, we also have added eight new titles in areas of increasing significance to today's youth. ADHD, or attention-deficit/hyperactivity disorder, and learning disorders are diagnosed with increasing frequency, and many students have observed or know of classmates receiving treatment for these conditions, even if they have not themselves received this diagnosis. Gambling is gaining currency in our culture, as casinos open and expand in many parts of the country, and the Internet offers easy access for this addictive behavior. Another consequence of our increasingly "online" society, unfortunately, is the presence of online predators. Environmental hazards represent yet another danger, and it is important to provide unbiased information about this topic to our youth. Suicide, which for many years has been a "silent epidemic," is now gaining recognition as a major public health problem throughout the life span, including the teenage and young adult years. We now also offer an overview of illness and disease in a volume that includes the major conditions of particular interest and concern to youth. In addition to illness, however, it is essential to emphasize health and its promotion, and this is especially apparent in the volumes on physical fitness and stress management.

It is our intent that each book serve as an accessible, authoritative resource to which young people can turn for accurate and meaningful answers to their specific questions. The series can help them research particular problems and provide an up-to-date evidence base. It is also designed with parents, teachers, and counselors in mind so that they have a reliable resource that they can share with youth who seek their guidance.

Finally, we have tried to provide unbiased facts rather than subjec-
tive opinions. Our goal is to help elevate the health of the public with
an emphasis on its most precious component—our youth. As young
people face the challenges of an increasingly complex world, we, as
educators, want them to be armed with the most powerful weapon
available—knowledge.

Robert N. Golden, M.D.
Fred L. Peterson, Ph.D.
General Editors

HOW TO
USE THIS BOOK

NOTE TO STUDENTS

Knowledge is power. By possessing knowledge you have the ability to make decisions, ask follow-up questions, or know where to go to obtain more information. In the world of health, that is power! That is the purpose of this book—to provide you the power you need to obtain unbiased, accurate information and *The Truth About Rape*.

Topics in each volume of The Truth About are arranged in alphabetical order, from A to Z. Each of these entries defines its topic and explains in detail the particular issue. At the end of most entries are cross–references to related topics. A list of all topics by letter can be found in the table of contents or at the back of the book in the index.

How have these books been compiled? First, the publisher worked with me to identify some of the country's leading authorities on key issues in health education. These individuals were asked to identify some of the major concerns that young people have about such topics. The writers read the literature, spoke with health experts, and incorporated their own life and professional experiences to pull together the most up-to-date information on health issues, particularly those of interest to adolescents and of concern in Healthy People 2010.

Throughout the alphabetical entries, the reader will find sidebars that separate Fact from Fiction. There are Question-and-Answer boxes that attempt to address the most common questions that youths ask about sensitive topics. In addition, readers will find special features called "Teens Speak"—case studies of teens with personal stories related to the topic in hand.

This may be one of the most important books you will ever read. Please share it with your friends, families, teachers, and classmates. Remember, you possess the power to control your future. One way to affect your course is through the acquisition of knowledge. Good luck and keep healthy.

NOTE TO LIBRARIANS

This book, along with the rest of The Truth About series, serves as a wonderful resource for young researchers. It contains a variety of facts, case studies, and further readings that the reader can use to help answer questions, formulate new questions, or determine where to go to find more information. Even though the topics may be considered delicate by some, don't be afraid to ask patrons if they have questions. Feel free to direct them to the appropriate sources, but do not press them if you encounter reluctance. The best we can do as educators is to let young people know that we are there when they need us.

Mark J. Kittleson, Ph.D.
Adviser to the First Edition

SOCIETY AND VICTIMS OF RAPE

Because sexual crimes can take many different forms, rape and other acts of sexual abuse are often referred to as sexual assault. Sexual assault is the most underreported of all serious crimes, according to a study by Edlin, Golanty, and McCormack, in 2000. It was estimated that in 1999, only 28.3 percent of sexual assaults in the United States were reported to the police. Statistics from the Department of Justice in 2005 show that things may have improved slightly, but even the newest estimates suggest that fewer than 40 percent of rapes and sexual assaults are reported to the police. Understandably, most people are sensitive about discussing their personal and sexual lives. In most societies, sexuality reveals intimate details that should be shared only by those we know well and who will not violate our trust.

Violating trust is a form of aggression, as are angry expressions, verbal insults, threats, physical harm, or sexual violence. In most cultures, aggression is encouraged. For example, to elevate their status, males are encouraged to act tough, take risks, strive for control, and exhibit power. They are discouraged from showing their emotions or appearing weak.

NEW IN THE REVISED EDITION

In this new edition of *The Truth About Rape*, all of the statistics have been revised to reflect the most recent information available. Key updates include new national statistics on rape and sexual assault from the Department of Justice, data that indicates that the incidence of sex crimes has gone down significantly over the past five years.

There is also new information about the role that technology might play in sexual assaults—from statistics on Internet predators to data on the effect that playing violent video games may have on a teenager's willingness to commit a rape or other violent crime. New graphs and new statistics on everything from the underreporting of sex offenses to the role of alcohol in sexual assaults on college campuses make this new volume a valuable tool for all teenagers who want or need to understand more about rape. One recent study of college students, for example, found that almost half of all women who had been raped were raped while they were incapacitated by alcohol or drugs that they had chosen to consume.

In addition, five new articles have been added to address areas that have recently come to light as being important to teens. One of the biggest modern concerns of young people has been the role of the Internet in sexual harassment and sexual assaults. Although the Internet is a wonderful and valuable tool, the very anonymity that many people find so freeing can also be a vehicle that sexual predators use to find—and pursue—their preferred victims. In the new entry "Internet Predators," readers can learn about what types of behaviors put individuals at risk on the Internet and how teenagers and others can keep themselves safe. They can also learn just how common different types of Internet sex crimes really are and what teens and their parents need to worry about online.

Another new entry, "Statutory Rape," focuses on the issue of a teenager's ability to consent to having sex. It explores how the legal age of consent varies from state to state and describes how two teenagers who decide to have sex with each other could, in some states, both end up in jail. Teenagers may be surprised to learn that, in seven states, if they choose to have sex with boyfriends or girlfriends who are only two years older than they, the age difference could lead to their partner's being arrested for statutory rape.

In "Rape Kits and Evidence Collection," readers will learn how physicians, nurses, and police collect evidence after a sexual assault. This is a very important chapter, because, if a teenager is ever sexually assaulted, knowing what to do and what not to do after a rape can make all the difference in seeing an attacker go to jail. The article also introduces a special group of nurses—sexual assault nurse examiners—who have been trained to make the process as efficient and stress-free as possible.

Two more new entries focus not only on statistics about sexual assault but also on how sexual assault affects, and is affected by, society. The entry "Female Rights" focuses on the role of women in society and how their freedoms and restrictions affect their risk of sexual assault. Covering everything from Take Back the Night rallies, which are designed to make the streets safer for women, to the role of religion in restricting women's sexual rights, freedoms, and options, "Female Rights" presents an overview of some of the major issues affecting women's sexual safety today.

Finally, "Rape and Society" takes the ideas of women's rights and discusses them in the context of human rights. In this article, teenagers will learn about gender-based violence and how assumptions about gender roles may make the people who live in some societies more accepting of rape. As cultural and societal perceptions may change, so may women's safety around the world. Rape is not just a crime against an individual; it is a pervasive problem that affects the public health of entire nations.

UNDERSTANDING RAPE

Historically, females have generally been considered inferior to men. In fact, in some cultures, children and women are considered a man's property and used according to a man's purposes. Even though women have served in the armed forces, held administrative positions, acted as government officials, and supported their families, the idea of male dominance has been continually reinforced. While the status of women in society has been elevated over the past few decades due to the importance of their social contributions, some people still feel that women, for example, should not take jobs away from men nor adopt their aspirations.

According to a 2009 report, many young men and women are exposed at an early age to sexually explicit content. Exposure to such content can make young people grow up with inappropriate views about what normal sexual behavior is and can lead to an increase in sexual risk taking. Even vulgar and obscene jokes can lead men to believe that seeing women as sexual "objects" is culturally acceptable. An earlier report found that by implying or portraying sexual acts of aggression, such jokes make it seem that sexual aggression is acceptable, or even desirable, behavior. In keeping with this stereotype, those who are aggressive toward others are often excused by parents, coaches, and others who advocate that "boys will be boys." Adults with this attitude convey the idea that it is acceptable to victimize others, thereby ignoring damage to the victims of aggression and their families, as well as the consequences to the perpetrators and their families.

In modern society, where people increasingly compete for the same resources, violent acts—including sexual crimes such as rape—are sometimes tolerated, justified, or overlooked by citizens, law enforcement personnel, and the legal system. As long as no one reports any harm, it is considered that no harm was done. When harm is reported, the **victim**, an unsuspecting person overpowered by a perpetrator, has to prove that he or she was taken advantage of and then detail the extent of the damage. He or she also has to prove that reasonable precautions were taken to prevent the situation and that the person who inflicted the harm is identified.

Violence—verbal or physical behavior carried out with the intent to harm, injure, or destroy someone or something—is used against people as a means of gaining power. Violence between two people is considered interpersonal violence and is a crime. Sexual assault and rape are types of interpersonal violence. Although not the same, they are similar. Neither sexual assault nor rape is about sex or passion. Both are crimes intended to inflict harm and are punishable by the criminal justice system.

THE DIFFERENCE BETWEEN SEXUAL ASSAULT AND RAPE

Assault is the threat—verbal or physical—of inflicting unwanted contact on a person, putting that person in danger or fear of danger. Sexual assault occurs when someone threatens or forces someone to have sexual contact against his or her will. Between a woman and a man, for example, if the woman is unwilling and does not give her permission, and the man forces his attention on her, the resulting contact is considered sexual assault. Sexual assault can range from unwanted sexual comments to fondling, molesting, forcing a victim to touch a perpetrator, or rape, traditionally when a man forces a woman—through coercion or deception—to have sexual intercourse against her will. In all situations, the victim is someone unwilling to have sexual contact with the other person but who is forced into the act because of a threat or actual harm. The object of sexual assault is to overpower, and sometimes humiliate, the victim. Both attempted sexual assaults and completed sexual assaults harm the victim in some way.

Rape is a type of sexual assault during which the mouth, vagina, or rectum is penetrated using objects or body parts. All rapes are felonies—major crimes punishable by at least one year in prison.

Different types of rape

There are many types of rape. Legally, a rape is considered one of three types: forcible rape, soft rape, and statutory rape. **Forcible rape** is sexual intercourse with a nonconsenting victim through the use or threat of force. Actual force does not need to be involved if the victim is afraid that harm will come to him or her. In soft rape, the perpetrator uses coercion in the form of physical pressure, psychological intimidation, or the threat of force in order to gain compliance from the victim. Statutory rape is sexual intercourse with a minor, a person who is under the legal age to give consent. A minor (in most states, someone under the age of 18) is considered to be incapable of understanding the act of sexual intercourse and therefore unable to freely give his or her consent.

The three categories of rape may occur as stranger rapes or acquaintance rapes. When most people think of rape, they think of stranger rape, where the victim is stalked, followed, and attacked by someone he or she did not know. Acquaintance rape is committed by someone the victim knows. In 2005, more than 75 percent of reported rapes were committed by someone the victim knew. Rape by an acquaintance can occur both at home and away, and these rapes are more likely than rapes committed by strangers because the victim usually trusts the assailant. "Soft" rapes are often acquaintance rapes.

Similar to acquaintance rape are date rape and partner rape. Date rape is rape that occurs when the victim and rapist are on a date. One study of rape on college campuses found that 13 percent of acquaintance rapes, and 35 percent of attempted acquaintance rapes, took place during a date. Another study based on the National Violence Against Women Survey found that 22 percent of female rape victims were raped by a current or former date, boyfriend, or girlfriend, and another 20 percent were raped by a spouse or ex-spouse. Although all states now recognize marital rape as a crime, in many states it is still considered a less serious offense, and the penalties are often not as severe as they are for other rapes. Still, the presence of marital rape laws at all is an enormous step forward. As recently as the mid-1970s, marital rape was legal in all of the 50 states. Although the idea is no longer accepted, women were once considered men's property, and a husband could have sexual intercourse with his wife whenever he wanted, even if she did not consent.

Rape is either attempted or completed. Legally, both attempted and completed rapes are considered sexual assault. Additionally, completed rapes can be called "simple" rapes or "aggravated" rapes. A simple rape is perpetrated by one person, without a physical beating or use of a weapon, by someone the victim knows. An aggravated rape involves physical beatings, weapons, multiple attackers, or strangers. Gang rape is one type of aggravated rape. When force is used, there is usually moderate to considerable bruising, tearing, and bleeding from the force. Many rapes result in injuries that require medical treatment even if no force is used.

Forced sexual activity can occur between men and women, men and men, women and women, married people, unmarried people, and adults and children. It can happen to infants, children, teenagers, adults, and elderly people. Most studies estimate that one in four women have been raped. As reported by Phillip Lenssen in 2000, most rape victims are young females. It is further estimated that nearly 29 percent of rape victims were under the age of 11, 32 percent between the ages of 11 and 17, and 22 percent between the ages of 18 and 24.

UNDERESTIMATING THE PROBLEM OF RAPE

Every year (according to authors Edlin, Golanty, McCormack, and Brown, in 2002) more than 100,000 forcible rapes are reported in the United States. In 2005 alone, the Department of Justice had reports of 70,000 rapes, 60,000 attempted rapes, and 60,000 sexual assaults. Many rapes are not reported because the victim is afraid, embarrassed, or in a state of disbelief or denial; thus this number is thought to be very low.

Underreporting: The stigma of rape

Rape is considered to be the most underreported of all violent crimes in the United States, according to Neft and Levine in 1997. In fact, according to the Bureau of Justice Statistics, from 1992 to 2000, only 26 percent of sexual assaults, 34 percent of attempted rapes, and

36 percent of completed rapes were reported to the police. Further, according to the National Crime Victimization Survey (NCVS), an annual average of 85,210 attempted and completed sexual assaults, 51,500 attempted rapes, and 64,080 completed rapes against persons aged 12 and older took place in 2004 and 2005. Overall, this is a significant improvement from previous years. The number of rapes and attempted rapes went down significantly, approximately 20 percent, from the preceding two-year period, while the number of sexual assaults went up only slightly, by just two percent. Looking over a longer period, the decline in sexual victimization is even clearer. In the years leading up to 2000, the average numbers were 152,680 sexual assaults, 209,230 attempted rapes, and 140,990 completed rapes—two to four times higher than in 2005. Also, as reported by the Bureau of Justice Statistics in 2005, most sexual assaults and rapes are committed against women. In fact, about 96 percent of all completed rapes, 80 percent of all attempted rapes, and 100 percent of all completed and attempted sexual assaults claimed female victims.

When a rape is reported, it is most likely reported by the victim. Victims of attempted or completed sexual assault or rape experience fear, denial, embarrassment, shame, guilt, anxiety. Researchers from the Bureau of Justice Statistics found that the most common reasons for a victim not to report a sexual assault or rape to police was that it was a "personal matter," fear of what might happen if they reported it, fear of what the police officer might think of them, and a desire to protect the perpetrator. The closer relationship the victim had with the perpetrator, the less the likelihood of the assault being reported. In fact, when the assailant was a current or former husband or boyfriend, 75–77 percent of sexual assaults, attempted rapes, and completed rapes were not reported. When the assailant was a stranger, the number of reports of sexual assaults, attempted rapes, and completed rapes increased.

In addition to the embarrassment or fear that may be associated with the reporting of a rape, no one wants to be "on trial" for a rape. Many victims feel that they, rather than the assailant, will be put on trial, particularly in the event of acquaintance rape. In addition to physical injuries, victims of rape often suffer from isolation, fear, shame, depression, and low self-esteem. Some suffer for years from post-traumatic stress disorder (PTSD), having recurring nightmares and other psychological disturbances requiring continued treatment.

The idea of having to relive the experience by telling it over and over again, and to risk judgment from authority figures, family members, significant others, and friends, is very difficult to bear.

Often, the perpetrator suffers fewer consequences than the victim. According to the Bureau of Justice Statistics report *Sex Offenses and Offenders* (1997), once an assault is reported, about half of all accused rapists are released before going to trial. Furthermore, in 2004, only 65 percent of convicted rapists went to prison. The average sentence was 10 years.

To help victims and law enforcement agencies arrest accused rapists, there are laws that permit communities to post pictures in local news-papers and post offices notifying residents of known sex offenders. The consequences of being accused and convicted of rape are severe.

Blaming the victim
In most cases, an accused rapist, abuser, or defendant never admits he or she has committed an act against someone or even that he or she committed a crime. Assailants may also deny ever physically or sexually hurting anyone. When a sexual assault is reported and the abuser identified, abusers may admit that they did it but try to make it sound as if the victim consented or "wanted it." The abuser might say that the victim "deserved it," placing the blame on the person who is hurt, rather than the one who did the abusing. Rapists usually do not care about the person they rape. They are consumed with issues of control, power, aggression, and self-gratification. Unfortunately, many believe that these traits are acceptable for males. Those who believe this are often surprised to find themselves charged and convicted for rape crimes. Those people usually are the ones misled by **rape myths**.

MYTHS
According to researchers Lonsway and Fitzgerald in 1994, myths about rape are accepted to deny or to justify male sexual aggres-sion against women. The more a culture supports the idea that men should be dominant and aggressive, the more it implies that women are inferior and sometimes worthy of aggression, as has been reported in 2002 by Murnen, Wright, and Kaluzny. Male sexual aggression is valued among males because it provides a way for them to prove their masculine identity and virility. According to

Symanski, Devlin, Chisler, and Vyse in 1993, males are expected to make sexual advances. Women are expected to be submissive. For these reasons, males are more likely to believe and perpetuate myths about rape. The more that myths about rape are accepted by men and women, the narrower the definition of rape becomes. Myths are perpetuated concerning what rape is, who a rapist is, and who rape victims are. In general, according to Johnson, Kuck, and Schander in a 1997 study, the myths include blaming the woman, excusing the man, and justifying rape between people who know each other.

Beliefs about rape vary according to the type of rape that occurred. According to Cowan in 2000, most people would not consider the victim to blame if the rape was perpetrated by a stranger. However, if the rapist is known to the victim, the woman is more likely to be blamed, especially if she was married to her assailant.

Some people believe that when someone is sexually assaulted or raped, the man or the woman somehow "asked for it" by dressing in revealing clothing, flirting, or showing signs of encouragement. When viewing a photograph of a rape victim in a short skirt, both men and women attributed the rape to the woman, as was reported in 1999 by Workman and Freeburn. Many men attribute more responsibility for a rape to the woman, whom they feel can be guilty of blame avoidance—blaming the rapist rather than one's own actions. In situations where men had been raped by men or women by women, victims blamed homosexual men and women even more than heterosexual women are blamed for the rapes against them, as reported by White, Robinson, and Kurpius in 2002. More traditional gender role attitudes often result in blaming victims as well as in increased negative attitudes toward gay men and lesbians. So do beliefs about proper behavior. A 2007 study by Sims, Noel, and Maisto found that both men and women were more likely to blame the victim of a rape if the victim was intoxicated when the rape occurred.

In one study by Syzmanski, Devlin, Chisler, and Vyse in 1993, males felt that about 50 percent of the time, women lied about being raped. One of the most harmful rape myths is that women manipulate men into having sex with them and then cry "rape." Another harmful myth is that women really want to be victims of aggression because they "like it."

Sometimes miscommunication is to blame for an act of sexual aggression. The more ambiguously one conveys the intention of sex, the more likely things will go wrong. Two types of ambiguous communication, according to Krahe, Scheinberger-Olwig, and Kolpin in 2000, are token resistance and **compliance**. Compliance is saying "yes" when you mean "no." In this situation, the person coerced into unwanted sexual activity submits. Token resistance is saying "no" when you mean "yes." The risk of sexual victimization and aggression in both cases is high.

Gender role expectations can be confusing. Rape can occur between people who know each other and are married to each other. Victims of rape can be wrongfully blamed for the crimes against them. The effects of rape can also be minimized by friends, family, medical professionals, and the police. For these and the numerous other reasons described, many rapes are not reported. As long as any type of rape is considered acceptable, members of society are to blame.

Again, although sexual assault and rape appear to be related to sex and sexuality, nothing could be further from the truth. Acts of sexual aggression are against the law. No one has the right to intimidate, threaten, or hurt another person. Some individuals gain a sense of power when they victimize another. These individuals are usually emotionally ill and need help. The majority of sexual aggressors and abusers were themselves abused as children. This exposure to violent acts of sexual aggression causes distorted thoughts and emotions that can lead to aggression toward others. And again, because sexual crimes are very personal, at times involving someone the victim knows, they are not always reported. Still, the number of sexual assaults and rapes that are reported indicate that the problem is prevalent and deserves serious attention. Citizens, parents, law enforcement personnel, teachers, and community leaders play essential roles in illuminating the problem and developing strategies to make communities and their citizens safer.

RISKY BUSINESS SELF-TEST: TRUE OR FALSE?

To identify whether your behavior or beliefs may put you at risk of being sexually assaulted, on a separate sheet of paper, write down whether you believe the following statements about rape are true or false:

Rape

_____ There is no permanent damage from rape.

_____ A society that does not seriously punish sexual harassment, a form of discrimination involving unwelcome sexual advances, will have no greater problems with rape than a society that does not tolerate it.

_____ When a woman does not yell, scream, or fight to avoid sexual intercourse, it technically is not rape.

_____ Rape victims who do not have hysterical reactions were not really raped.

_____ Someone who is drunk or high can still make informed decisions about having sex.

_____ Men cannot be raped.

_____ Children who have been sexually abused have not been raped.

_____ Anyone who is raped is responsible for his or her own rape.

_____ Women are the only victims of rape.

_____ Rape victims are young, attractive, financially well-off, and white.

Stranger rape

_____ Most sexual assaults occur on impulse.

_____ A rapist is most likely to be from an undereducated and poor background.

_____ A rapist is sexually deprived and needs to rape for sexual gratification.

_____ Women secretly want to be raped.

_____ Women who are "easy" or "loose" cannot be raped because they want to have sex with any man.

_____ Rapists can only be strangers.

Date rape

_____ When a woman or man invites someone into their home to have coffee, it means that they want to have sex.

_____ Women claim they have been raped to "get back" at a man.

_____ When a woman on a date refuses to have sex, she is flirting and really wants to have sex; therefore, the man should insist.

_____ When there are no bruises, tears, or other physical injuries, unwanted sexual intercourse is not considered rape.

_____ Rape is just "rough sex" that gets out of control.

In fact, *all* of the above statements are myths, not true.

See also: Abusive Sexual Behavior; Female Rights; Law and Rape, The; Rape and Society; Sexual Assault, Types of; Stigma of Rape; Victims of Rape: Female; Victims of Rape: Male

A-TO-Z ENTRIES

■ ABORTION LAWS
See: Law and Rape, The

■ ABUSIVE SEXUAL BEHAVIOR
Abusive sexual behavior is sexual misconduct that ranges from derogatory, demeaning, contemptuous, or damaging to brutal, cruel, exploitative, painful, or violent. Abusive sexual behavior includes sexual contact or sexual attention obtained through force, threats, bribes, **manipulation**, pressure, tricks, or violence.

SOCIAL INFLUENCES
Societal attitudes toward the role of women in society, sexual behavior, and violence may all influence the occurrence and perception of abusive sexual behavior. Some experts argue that the social dynamic between men and women is a source of violent crimes against women and that resocialization can be used as a prevention tool. In other words, teaching people to have improved attitudes toward women and their place in society can help prevent abusive relationships from occurring or persisting. As stereotypical portrayals of women in the media are often sources of negative attitudes toward women, a change in image can positively influence a change in behavior.

Fact Or Fiction?

Rapists tend to be uneducated and work in low-paying jobs.

The Facts: Rapists come from all backgrounds. They can be highly educated and work in professional jobs. Others may in fact be poorly educated or unemployed. There is no way to tell based on the amount of money someone has, or by the job that he or she holds, whether or not that person is capable of committing a sexual assault.

A 2005 study of Israeli students found that individuals with more traditional, as opposed to egalitarian, beliefs about gender roles were less likely to perceive a sexual assault incident as severe. Such attitudes were more common among men than women, but the association was found across both genders. This type of belief is related to the results of the 1993 article "Profiling the Rapist: Predictions of Dangerousness," in which William Glaser found that rapists tended to regard women as objects existing only for their gratification rather than as individuals. Similarly, in her article "When Words Are Not Enough: The Search for the Effect of Pornography on Abused Women," Janet Hinson Shope correlates the use of **pornography**, which is media of no literary or artistic value other than to stimulate sexual desire, with sexual abuse in relationships. The use of pornography may be related to this vision of women as sex objects. These and other social influences can cause rapists to confuse what is ordinarily an act of love with power, violence, and control.

DEFICIENT SOCIAL SKILLS

Some research, much of which is based on the work of clinical psychologists Abel, Blanchard, and Becker from the mid-1970s, suggests that in a high percentage of rape cases (including domestic, date, and gang rape), the rapist seeks to bolster a poor self-image by attacking someone who is perceived as weaker. In these rape cases, the attacker is usually male and tends to have low intelligence and few social skills combined with a profound sense of his own inferiority in his dealings with others. A deep-seated fear of women is more common than a feeling of superiority, and this may lie in early failure to make successful relationships.

The psychologists found that many of the sex offenders they treated had poor heterosocial skills—that is, they lacked the social skills necessary to function with individuals of the opposite sex. Their observations led to a large body of research that examined the social and heterosocial competence of rapists and child molesters.

In 1977, the initial studies of Barlow and others suggested that rape and the sexual abuse of children are sexual **deviations** that result, in part, from an inability to establish normal sexual relationships. Rape was identified by Freund in 1988 as a "courtship disorder," or an inability to perform normally in a courtship situation. However, further research has indicated that these characterizations might only apply to a minority of rapists who develop a preference for rape over consensual intercourse.

DID YOU KNOW?

Correlation Between Those Abused as Juveniles and Future Crime

Individuals who were abused as adolescents are more than twice as likely to be arrested or commit a violent offence during young adulthood.

Source: Smith, C. A. et al. (2005) "Adolescent Maltreatment and Its Impact on Young Adult Antisocial Behavior" *Child Abuse & Neglect* 29, no. 10: 1,099–1,119.

A 2008 study published in *Clinical Psychology Review* noted that men who are more likely to commit rape tend to perceive women as being more sexually interested in them than do other men. This inability to correctly perceive a woman's sexual intention may be related to the low levels of heterosocial competence that have also been reported in rapists and child molesters. Heterosocial competence is the ability to competently interact with members of the opposite sex. The authors of the 2003 *Journal of Sex Research* survey concluded that rapists showed lower heterosocial competence than nonrapists but that child molesters are even more deficient in their ability to interact with members of the opposite sex than rapists.

PSYCHOLOGICAL IMPAIRMENTS

Defining the psychological profile of a violent criminal is difficult. The rapist who attacks a stranger may be psychologically different from a pedophile or a date rapist. For date or acquaintance rape, some simple warning signs exist that indicate potential for violence against women. Be aware and conscious of the following:

- Someone who is overly aggressive in his daily behavior
- A man who does not respect your feelings or wishes
- A man who regularly invades your body space or is too "touchy-feely"
- A man who is overtly or verbally hostile to women
- A man who physically or sexually comes on too strong

- A man who makes lewd, demeaning comments about women, especially of a sexual nature

- A man who shows that he feels he must control your behavior or treats you as his property

- A man who expresses archaic or wrong ideas about women, such as "they're sex objects," or "nice girls don't get raped"

A man may not exhibit any of these behaviors early in a relationship but may still be a date rapist. If something feels wrong, women should trust their instincts.

The Federal Bureau of Investigation (FBI) classifies rapists into four groups. According to the agency, 44 percent of rapists seek to gain power and control and assert their sexuality. They pick on those who seem most vulnerable and use trickery, manipulation, intimidation, verbal abuse, and isolation to gain access to their prey.

A second group commits sexual assaults in order to retaliate for real or imagined pain against men, women, or both. The assailants in this type of rape also hope to gain power and control and reassure themselves of their own sexuality. Many use extreme physical force to overpower their victims.

The third group of rapists are acting out their fantasies. Some of these men expect to find someone who will love what they have to offer. They are unable to establish a relationship with a woman through ordinary means, but they want to feel reassured that they are sexually valued. They believe that the woman really wants to be raped. Others of this type are seeking revenge for real or imagined suffering caused by the victim or the victim's gender. They feel they have lost power to the victim or to someone of the same gender, often their mothers. They use rape to restore their power through domination, making the victim feel powerless. In doing so, they are reassured of their power. Both types of rapists in this group gain access to their victims through intimidation, verbal abuse, and manipulation.

A very small number of rapists are excited by watching a victim suffer. This fourth type of rapist is extremely violent and death of the victim may result.

HEREDITY AND ENVIRONMENTAL INFLUENCES

Although most men who undergo traumatic experiences as children do not grow up to be rapists, research suggests that many offenders were once victims of some kind of abuse—if not of sexual abuse, then at least of social and emotional deprivation. However, not all abused children grow up to be abusers, and not all rapists were abused as children. As a result, it cannot be said that child abuse causes sexual violence in adults.

Rapists come from every economic background, every profession, and every culture. Although they tend to lack social skills, they may be otherwise indistinguishable from anyone else. There is no direct evidence that sexually abusive tendencies are inherited. Although children who grow up in violent households are more likely to become violent adults, it remains unclear how much their behavior is the result of **heredity** and how much is the result of environmental exposure, or learning by watching.

See also: Children and Rape; Date Rape; Rape Within Abusive Relationships; Sexual Harassment; Sexual Violence and Children

FURTHER READING

Feuereisen, Patti. *Invisible Girls: The Truth About Sexual Abuse—A Book for Teen Girls, Young Women, and Everyone Who Cares About Them.* New York: Seal Press, 2005.

Rudman, Laurie A., and Peter Glick. *The Social Psychology of Gender: How Power and Intimacy Shape Gender Relations.* New York: The Guilford Press, 2008.

ACQUAINTANCE RAPE

See: Date Rape

ALCOHOL AND RAPE

See: Drugs, Alcohol, and Rape; Educating the Community; Gang Rape; Prevention of Rape: Being Proactive

CHILDREN AND RAPE

Children and rape involves the impact of sexual assaults—including incest, or sexual intercourse between family members who are not husband and wife—on juveniles (individuals under the age of 18).

Juvenile Victims of Sexual Abuse

Approximately one-fifth of all juvenile victims of sexual abuse in the United States are children under the age of 12.

Source: U.S. Department of Health and Human Services, Administration on Children, Youth and Families. *Child Maltreatment*, 2006.

In 2006, more than 78,000 juveniles were victims of sexual abuse, according to the U.S. Department of Health and Human Services. Approximately 11 percent of those children were under the age of eight, and a similar number were between the ages of eight and 11. Many of the **assailants** were also children. In fact, one study reported about 40 percent of offenders who victimized children under the age of six were juveniles themselves.

A Bureau of Justice Statistics study from 2000 found that 93 percent of the victims of juvenile sexual assault knew their attackers, meaning family members committed 34 percent of the attacks, and acquaintances were responsible for 59 percent. Only 7 percent of the perpetrators were strangers to the victim. All attackers used or threatened to use force when committing a criminal sexual act.

Q & A

Question: Are teenagers at higher risk for sexual assault?

Answer: Yes. Teens ages 16–19 were three and one-half times more likely than the general population to be victims of rape, attempted rape, or sexual assault, according to the National Crime Victimization Survey.

ENCOURAGING NONVIOLENT BEHAVIOR

The world is full of violence, and children are exposed to violence daily on television, in movies, and in video games. Children often face the fear of violence at school or in their neighborhood. The role of parents and guardians is to protect children as well as to raise them to be nonviolent individuals.

One of the main tenets for raising nonviolent children is to listen to them and respect them. It is also important to encourage children to express their feelings through words rather than violent action. If parents model respectful behavior and treat their child with respect, they will have a child who respects himself or herself as well as others.

When disagreements arise in a family, members need to help explore alternatives. For example, family meetings can be helpful in working out long-term disputes and avoiding future misunderstandings. Members who feel like they count, and who are given responsibility in the family, are less likely to act out in inappropriate ways.

Childhood exposure to violent media has been shown to be associated with violent behaviors later in life. A large 2009 study of American youth found that a preference for violent media was associated not only with violent behavior in adulthood but also with having a callous attitude toward others. This is one reason why monitoring exposure to violence in the media can also help young family members to grow up to be nonviolent adults. A study published in the *Journal of Developmental Psychology* found that childhood watching of TV violence led to an increase in aggressive adult behavior, including spousal abuse and other criminal offenses, regardless of how the adults behaved as children. Children process information visually, and visual images have a much greater emotional impact than words, therefore it is not surprising that children may be profoundly impacted by what they see. They may be even more affected by what they do. Numerous studies in a special January 2004 video game issue of the *Journal of Adolescence* found that video games, in particular, were associated with children becoming not only desensitized to violence but also more aggressive in both their actions and their self-identity. Acting out violent behaviors, such as murder and rape, may actually make them seem, in some way, more emotionally acceptable.

Adults and young adults must be careful to not act violently in front of younger siblings or children. This includes not yelling at others or expressing one's anger loudly or irrationally. In fact, one should never act violently toward others. If a child in your family acts aggressively, teach him or her more appropriate methods of expressing frustration or anger.

PREVENTION STRATEGIES FOR CHILDREN

According to the National Center for Missing and Exploited Children, there are a number of strategies that parents, guardians, and older siblings can take to minimize the risk that a child will become a victim. These strategies include:

- Listening to children. Pay attention if they say they do not want to go somewhere or be with someone.
- Encouraging open communication with children or younger siblings
- Teaching children that they have the right to say no if anyone touches them or talks to them in an inappropriate manner. Make sure children know that any touch that is unwelcome, uncomfortable, or confusing is not okay.
- Being aware of any changes, even small ones, in a child's behavior or attitude
- Noticing when someone starts paying a lot of attention to a child in your family or giving him or her gifts
- Striving to stay nonconfrontational, nonjudgmental, and calm if a child confides in you
- Screening all babysitters and caregivers. Check references with other families. Drop in unexpectedly to see what is happening. Ask children about the caregiver and listen to the responses. If your state has a public registry of sexual predators or **pedophiles**, check to see if the caregiver has a prior criminal history.
- Providing supervision of a child's computer use. Know with whom she or he is communicating.
- Practicing and openly discussing basic safety skills with the children in your family

Fact Or Fiction?

Most children who are sexually abused are girls.

The Facts: According to a 1995 study on child maltreatment that was conducted by the Department of Health and Human Services Administration for Children and Families, local child protective service agencies identi-fied 126,000 children who were victims of either substantiated or indi-cated sexual abuse. Of these, 75 percent were girls.

It is important that children in a family know that they can always come to the adults to talk about anything. Many children keep quiet about abuse, including rape. They are usually frightened or intimi-dated by the offender, or they may think that no one will believe them or that they will somehow be blamed. The more open the lines of communication are within families, the more likely it is that a sexually abused child or teen will tell someone what is happening. Once a family member knows about the abuse, he or she should try to stop it before it becomes a recurring problem. The goal of sharing is to get your child or sibling help as soon as possible. It is important that children understand that it is the adult who is wrong in these situations and that the child victim is not to blame.

Fact Or Fiction?

Most children who are sexually abused are in elementary school or younger.

The Facts: According to the 2006 report on Child Maltreatment from the Department of Health and Human Services Administration on Children, Youth and Families, local child protective service agencies identified 78,000 children who were victims of sexual abuse. Approximately 22 per-cent of them were under the age of 12.

TEENS AND RAPE

Sexual intercourse between an adult and a person under the "age of consent" (usually under 18) is called statutory rape. Like children, teens are often victims too, and they are particularly susceptible to sexual violence. According to a 1996 study conducted by the Alan Guttmacher Institute, seven in 10 women who had sex before age 14, and six in 10 of those who had sex before age 15, report that it was involuntary, or without their consent. Overall, according to the 2005 National Crime Victimization Survey, teens 16–19 years of age were more than three times more likely than the general population to be victims of rape, attempted rape, or sexual assault. Although 90 percent of rapes are perpetrated on women or girls, boys and men are also at risk.

In the case of date rape or acquaintance rape (nonconsensual sex between people who have a social dating relationship), victims are often confused about whether what they experienced was rape or not. A victim may not be sure that she did not give her consent somehow, even if she knows she did not want to have sex. The perpetrator often feels he is "entitled" to sex.

Both attitudes are incorrect. Unless sex is fully consensual for both parties, it can be classified as rape. No one can force you to have sex against your will—if you say no, and the person has sex with you anyway, it is rape. Similarly, if you continue to have sex with someone after that person has said no or made it clear that she is uncomfortable or unhappy with your attention, this is rape.

If you are raped on a date, it is important not to blame yourself. It is the fault of the rapist. You do not have to accept any level of violence. When dating, it helps to keep the following guidelines in mind:

- Know your wishes, limits, and values, and clearly communicate them to your dates.
- Pay attention if your date does not respect your limits and wishes or if your date's behavior does not seem appropriate. Before things get out of control, you might want to think about leaving under these circumstances.
- Trust your feelings and intuition; if you are feeling pressured into sex, it is not right. Both boys and girls have the right to say "no."
- Be assertive and act immediately if your limits are reached—even if it means making a scene.
- Understand that it is never too late to say "no" and never too late to hear "no."

See also: Date Rape; Help and Support; Internet Predators; Statutory Rape; Sexual Violence and Children

FURTHER READING

Feuereisen, Patti. *Invisible Girls: The Truth About Sexual Abuse—A Book for Teen Girls, Young Women, and Everyone Who Cares About Them.* New York: Seal Press, 2005.

Mather, Cynthia L. *How Long Does It Hurt: A Guide to Recovering from Incest and Sexual Abuse for Teenagers, Their Friends, and Their Families.* San Francisco: Jossey-Bass, 2004.

■ DATE RAPE

Date rape is forced sexual contact (oral, vaginal, or anal) that occurs in a dating relationship. Date rape is also known as **acquaintance rape**, which is rape by an assailant who is known to the victim. According to FBI figures, more than 80 percent of all rapes are acquaintance rapes, and more than 55 percent of acquaintance rapes occur on dates. The assailant is often a boyfriend or girlfriend but may also be a neighbor, coworker, classmate, family friend, teacher, relative, tutor, mentor, religious leader, or camp counselor.

Date rape, like other kinds of rape, is a felony, a crime punishable with a prison term that can range from one to 25 years. In the eyes of the law, date rape is as serious a crime as rape by a stranger. It is a crime that occurs in both heterosexual and homosexual (same-sex) relationships. Although most perpetrators are male and most victims are female, women can also be assailants and men victims. Date rape is the most common type of rape among young people.

The assailants in a date rape rarely use a weapon. Instead, they rely on threats, coercion, physical strength, or authority to intimidate or overpower their victims. Victims of acquaintance rape often report that they initially trusted and liked their assailant, not recognizing the intent to rape until it was too late to get help.

Some date rapes are also considered statutory rapes. A **statutory rape** is sexual intercourse with an individual who state laws determine to be too young to give his or her consent. Based on the idea that children do not fully understand the consequences of a sexual relationship, the **age of consent** varies by state. In some states, the age of consent is as young as 14. In most, it is between 16 and 18 years of age. Even if the underage person agrees to have sex, his or her older partner can be charged and prosecuted for statutory rape.

HOW COMMON IS DATE RAPE?

No one knows for certain how frequently date rape occurs because victims are often reluctant to report the crime to the police or other authorities. Researchers Mary P. Koss and Mary R. Harvey report that among the more than 6,000 college students they surveyed in a 1991 study, 50 percent of victims never reported an acquaintance rape to the police. Another report based on the National Violence Against Women Survey found that fewer than 10 percent of individuals who were sexually assaulted by someone they knew reported the assault to the police. The percentage reporting is three

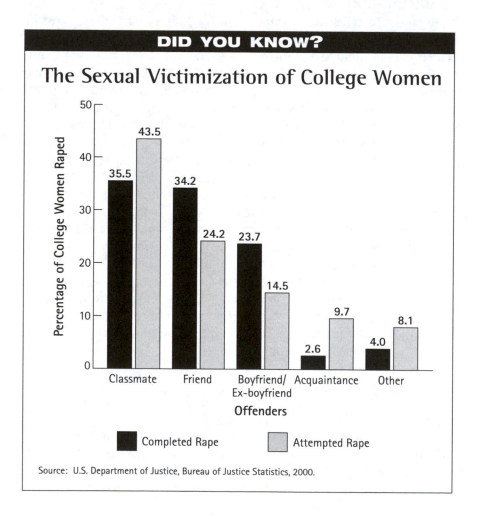

DID YOU KNOW?

The Sexual Victimization of College Women

Percentage of College Women Raped

- Classmate: 35.5 (Completed Rape), 43.5 (Attempted Rape)
- Friend: 34.2 (Completed Rape), 24.2 (Attempted Rape)
- Boyfriend/Ex-boyfriend: 23.7 (Completed Rape), 14.5 (Attempted Rape)
- Acquaintance: 2.6 (Completed Rape), 9.7 (Attempted Rape)
- Other: 4.0 (Completed Rape), 8.1 (Attempted Rape)

Offenders

■ Completed Rape   □ Attempted Rape

Source: U.S. Department of Justice, Bureau of Justice Statistics, 2000.

times higher in people who were sexually assaulted by a stranger. Additionally, in November 1998, researchers V. I. Rickett and C. M. Wieman reported in the *Journal of Pediatric and Adolescent Gynecology* that the frequency of date rape ranges from 20 percent to 68 percent among adolescent girls and 13 percent to 27 percent among college-age women.

That study and others like it also show that date rape is a serious problem among high school and college students. A 2007 study on campus sexual assault by the National Institute of Justice found that 15 percent of female undergraduates had been the victims of a rape or attempted rape before starting college, and another 19 percent had been victimized while on campus. At the time of the assaults, almost half of the women who were the victims of a completed assault on campus were incapacitated by alcohol or drugs that they had chosen to consume. A much smaller number of sexual assault victims were forcibly assaulted or drugged by their attackers. Of the women who were incapacitated by drugs or alcohol at the time of the assault, more than 80 percent either knew their attackers or had at least seen them on campus. In fact, 17 percent of them were on dates with their attackers at the time that the rape occurred, and almost 30 percent of the attackers were fraternity members. When it came to forcible rapes, 76 percent of the women were at least familiar with their attacker, 19 percent were on a date with their rapist at the time of the attack, and 14 percent of the attackers were fraternity members.

High school students are also affected. A study of 2,000 eighth- and ninth-grade students published in the *American Journal of Preventive Medicine* indicated that nearly 11 percent of these students were victims of an act of sexual violence. The 2003 Youth Risk Behavioral Surveillance Survey (YRBS) found that 12 percent of high school girls and 6 percent of high school boys had been forced to have sex at least once in their lifetime. Also, the Minnesota Student Survey, a 1998 study of more than 81,000 students in the ninth and 12th grades, revealed that 9 percent of girls and 6 percent of boys had experienced violence, including rape, in a dating relationship. The rate of dating violence is not notably decreasing over time. The 2003 YRBS also found that approximately 9 percent of both high school girls and boys had experienced physical violence in a dating relationship.

FACTORS THAT CONTRIBUTE TO DATE RAPE

Although each act of rape may have numerous causes, a variety of factors contribute to the frequency of date rapes among young people. Those factors include the attitudes and behaviors of the perpetrators as well as those of society in general.

The assailant

What prompts someone to rape a date, a friend, or other acquaintance? While psychologists have devised no single profile of a person likely to commit a rape, they have identified characteristics many assailants share. These include:

- An inclination toward violence in attempts to solve problems
- Aggressiveness in intimate relationships
- A tendency to be overly demanding of partners.

An alarming element of concern to researchers is their finding that, in fact, many perpetrators often do not consider themselves rapists. In 1985, Mary Koss, then a professor of psychology at Kent State University, surveyed approximately 7,000 students on 32 college campuses and found that one in every 12 men admitted to having forced a woman to have intercourse (rape) or tried to force a woman to have intercourse (attempted rape) through physical force or coercion. Although these men acknowledged they used force or coercion, virtually none of them identified themselves as rapists. Similarly, only 57 percent of their victims labeled the experience as rape; the other 43 percent did not even acknowledge to themselves that they had been raped. A smaller study, "A Comparison of Men Who Committed Different Types of Sexual Assault in a Community Sample," completed in 2007, found that 64 percent of the men in the study population had committed some form of sexual assault since the age of 14. Their crimes ranged from coercing a woman into having sex to forcible rape.

Myths and misinformation about date rape

The attitudes of both the assailants and their victims were shaped at least in part by the values and beliefs of the society in which they live. Researchers have found that a variety of myths and mistaken beliefs may explain why both men and women have difficulty identifying a date or acquaintance rape. Those myths include:

- "Maybe" means "yes."
- If a woman has previously been sexually active, she will probably be willing to have sex with other men.
- If a woman agrees to any sexual contact, including kissing or fondling, she has agreed to "go all the way."
- If a woman has had sex with a man once, she will be willing to have sex again.
- Buying dinner or gifts entitles a man to have sex with his date.
- Date rape is the result of miscommunication.
- Rape happens only when a stranger forces a woman to have sexual intercourse.
- Rape occurs only when there is physical violence or a physical struggle.

Q & A

Question: I've heard people say that it is never a girl's fault if she is raped. But isn't she asking for sex if she wears see-through tops or tight clothes that show off her body?

Answer: The way people dress does not invite rape. Rape and other sexual assaults are acts of violence. Victims are often selected because they appear vulnerable.

These myths are dangerous because they shift responsibility for a rape from the assailant to the victim. To the extent that victims of date rape share those mistaken beliefs, they are less likely to resist forcefully and clearly. Those attitudes can also hinder the criminal justice system. Too often, juries focus on a victim's morals, lifestyle, and dress rather than the offender's actions. The truth is, a person has the right to say "no" to sex at any time, regardless of how the victim looks or behaves or whether the couple has had sex in the past.

Fact Or Fiction?

If a girl visits a date's bedroom, it's partly her fault if she is raped.

The Facts: According to the federal government's Office on Violence Against Women, the victim is never responsible for the rape. It makes no difference where a rape occurs. Forcing sex on a person without their consent is a sexual assault.

Alcohol and drugs

A date rape is more likely to occur when alcohol or drugs are present. According to researcher Mary P. Koss in *Rape and Sexual Assault* (Vol. 2), 75 percent of male college students and 55 percent of female students who were involved in a date rape had been drinking or taking drugs at the time the rape occurred. In a 2007 study by the National Institute of Justice, researchers also found that almost half of all rapes that took place on campus were attacks on women who were incapacitated by alcohol or drugs. Interestingly, many women who were assaulted did not necessarily think a crime had taken place, and this viewpoint was highly affected by whether or not substance use was involved in the attack. Of the women who, by their own testimony, were raped, only 65 percent of women who were forcibly raped, and 38 percent of women who were raped while incapacitated by drugs or alcohol, actually considered the assault to be rape.

Alcohol and drugs are dangerous because they interfere with thinking and reasoning ability. They also make it harder to communicate clearly.

Alcohol is the most commonly abused substance in date rapes among all age groups. A Harvard School of Public Health study published in 2004 states that among college women who had been raped in the previous year, 72 percent were so intoxicated that they were not able to agree to sex or to emphatically refuse it.

Experts warn teens to be wary of a friend or acquaintance who pushes alcohol or drugs. Some assailants encourage their victims to get high, drowsy, or even unconscious so that they will not be able to resist. Some offenders even put drugs into a victim's beverage without his or her knowledge.

Obviously, it is a crime to use illegal drugs. Giving another person drugs of any kind without his or her consent is also a crime. And it is also a crime to have sex with someone who is physically unable to give consent. According to a 2004 report issued by the National Institute on Drug Abuse, the drugs most commonly used in a date rape are GHB (gamma hydroxybutyrate) and Rohypnol (flunitrazepam). A 2003 Mayo Clinic report states that more than 20 other drugs are also used, including Klonopin (clonazepam), Ketalan (ketamine), Ativan (lorazepam), and Xanax (alprazolam). Benadryl, an antihistamine sold over the counter, is also sometimes used.

With the exception of Benadryl, these drugs depress the central nervous system. They have a sedative effect—that is, they relax the user and make him or her feel drowsy by decreasing the heart rate and the breathing rate. They also weaken the muscles. These drugs are especially dangerous when combined with alcohol, which increases the drugs' potency, causing them to have a more powerful effect on the body.

Date rape drugs are likely to appear at clubs, house parties, sporting events, or at casual gatherings. GHB, also known as liquid ecstasy, scoop, easy lay, vita-G, and Georgia Home Boy, is colorless, tasteless, and odorless. It can be added to a drink without the victim being aware of it. A small amount of GHB tends to make a person very drowsy. In higher, more dangerous amounts, the drug can cause seizures and coma. It is particularly dangerous when combined with alcohol.

Rohypnol, sometimes known as roofies, rophies, roach, and rope, acts very much like GHB. Although it is not as popular as it was during the 1990s, it is still in use. It, too, cannot be detected when added to drinks. Rohypnol can also cause amnesia. A person under the influence of Rohypnol is unlikely to recall what occurred while the drug was in his or her body.

Psychologists and other counselors suggest that individuals take special precautions at parties and other gatherings. Those precautions include:

- Watching while a beverage is poured or accepting drinks only from bottles or cans that partygoers have opened for themselves
- Never leaving a beverage unattended

- Avoiding alcohol or drugs while on a date
- Calling a friend if feeling sick or dizzy after drinking and, if necessary, calling 911

PREVENTING DATE RAPE

There is no sure way to prevent a rape. However, people can do many things to decrease the odds of becoming a victim or a perpetrator. Some experts suggest that women:

- Meet in public places on the first few dates with someone they don't know well
- Do not go to a date's car or home or to their own home if they will be alone there
- Plan to take public transportation home or arrange to have someone they know pick them up after a date
- Set sexual limits and make their dates aware of those limits
- Clearly communicate their expectations to their dates
- Stay sober. It is easier to be in control of a situation when one is not under the influence of alcohol or drugs.
- Trust their instincts. If a woman feels uneasy or threatened in a situation, she should get away as quickly as possible. There is no need to explain or find an excuse to leave if one feels uncomfortable.

Experts suggest that men can prevent date rape by:

- Never forcing a woman to have sex even if she said yes at first
- Staying sober
- Not assuming that a woman's intoxication or sexual history has any bearing on her right to say no
- Not supposing that they know what a woman wants or that she knows what a man wants. A successful relationship is built on communication. If a man feels he is getting a mixed message, he should speak up and ask the woman to clarify what she wants.

■ Communicating with other men if they are over-stepping bounds

AID FOR VICTIMS OF DATE RAPE

Date rape victims experience many of the same emotions after the assault as victims of other forms of sexual violence. They, too, feel frightened, ashamed, depressed, embarrassed, and humiliated. However, victims of date rape also face problems that are specific to their victimization. Because the rapist is often someone they knew or even socialized with, victims often have to face their assailant after the rape.

Victims of date rape often feel that they were to blame in some way for the rape or that they could have prevented it. The truth is, no victim is ever to blame for being raped. The rapist is always the one at fault.

Victims of a date rape also experience **trauma**, an emotional and physical shock. That trauma is as severe as the one experienced by someone raped by a stranger. About one-third of all rape victims suffer from rape-related post-traumatic stress disorder (PTSD), a condition that often includes sleeping and eating disorders, nervousness, fatigue, withdrawal from society, and distrust of others. Many victims suffer from one or several of these symptoms. Some are affected for many years.

If you or someone you know is a victim of a date rape, psychologists and other health-care professionals suggest the following:

■ Go to a friend's place. If there is no one to go to, call someone you can talk to, no matter how late it is.

■ Get medical attention. Do not shower, bathe, or change your clothing first. Go to a hospital or health center to be examined and treated for possible venereal disease. There may also be internal injuries. If you decide to press charges, physical specimens collected soon after the rape may be valuable evidence.

■ Report the attack even if you do not plan to file charges. Someone who has raped once is likely to rape again. If you turn the rapist in, you may save someone else from being attacked.

■ Get help and support. You have been through a trauma and need help to deal with the situation and your feelings. People who seek counseling get over their experiences faster and with fewer lasting effects than those who do not get help.

TEENS SPEAK

I Was Raped on a Date

Last year, Jerry, a popular guy on the basketball team, sat beside me in geometry class. We wrote funny notes to each other. One day he asked me to go to a party with him.

The night of the party we drove with a bunch of kids to the house of one of Jerry's friends. In the car he sat close to me and kept putting his hands all over me and kissing me hard on the mouth. At one point he said he wanted to "get really close to me," and I said "okay." I knew he meant sex. I don't know why I agreed to it. I guess I thought it was expected of me. I didn't want to have sex with him.

At the party, there was beer and someone was passing around bottles of Tequila. I could see that Jerry was getting drunk. I had three beers to try to calm myself down. A couple of hours later, Jerry put his arm around me and steered me out to the backyard. He pulled me down and started to kiss me and pull off my clothes. I felt so confused I didn't know what to do. I told him to stop and kept pushing him away, but he said that I told him that I wanted to have sex.

I felt bad, because I had sort of told him I would. I began to doubt myself. Was I right to refuse to have sex? I was so tired from the beer, and I felt so upset that I couldn't think straight. Before I knew what was happening, he raped me.

After it happened, I felt terrible. I felt it was my fault. I told my best friend who urged me to tell my counselor at school. I was so desperate that I went to see her. I was relieved that she tried to help me. It helped me make some decisions about what I wanted to do next.

DID YOU KNOW?

Alcohol Use by Those Convicted of Rape and Sexual Assault

According to surveys of probationers and local, state, and federal prisoners:

- 32 percent of adults on probation who had been convicted of sexual assault were drinking at the time of the rape.
- 32 percent of convicted rapists in local jails were drinking at the time of the offense.
- 36 percent of convicted rapists in state prisons were drinking at the time of the offense.
- 27 percent of convicted rapists in federal prisons were drinking at the time of the rape.

Source: Alcohol and Crime, National Symposium on Alcohol Abuse and Crime, U.S. Department of Justice, 1998.

A 1993 report by the Senate Judiciary Committee noted that 71 percent of rape victims fear their families will find out that they have been sexually assaulted; 69 percent worry that people will think it was their fault; 50 percent worry that their names will appear in the media. Other reasons for not reporting a rape are possibly more disturbing. A 2002 report by the U.S. Department of Justice, in which researchers looked at 10 years of data on rape, injury, and reporting, found that in cases of rape, 23 percent of victims did not report the crime because it was a personal matter; 16 percent of victims did not report because of a fear of reprisal; and 6 percent did not report because they thought that the police might be biased. In cases of attempted rape, however, almost 10 percent of women did not report the crime because they wanted to protect the offender.

These numbers seem to remain consistent over time. In 2005, 22 percent of sexual assault victims told the Department of Justice that they did not report their crime to the police because it was a private or personal matter. For these reasons and more, many rape victims never reach out for services or assistance. Fewer than half of rape victims report the crime to the police, according to 2005 victimization statistics from the Department of Justice, and earlier research suggests that their estimates may actually be high. A 1992 study from the National Center for Victims of Crime & Victims Research and Treatment found that only 16 percent of victims reported the crime to the police. Sadly, even when victims do step forward and report, they are often not believed.

See also: Drugs, Alcohol, and Rape; Help and Support; Prevention of Rape: Being Proactive; Prevention of Rape: Being Reactive; Rape Within Abusive Relationships; Sexual Assault, Types of; Statutory Rape; Victims of Rape: Female; Victims of Rape: Male

FURTHER READING

Gunton, Sharon. *Date and Acquaintance Rape.* Social Issues Firsthand. New York: Greenhaven Press, 2009.

Landau, Elaine. *Date Violence.* Danbury, Conn.: Childrens Press, 2005.

McGregor, Joan. *Is It Rape? On Acquaintance Rape and Taking Women's Consent Seriously.* Burlington, Vt.: Ashgate Publishing, 2005.

White, Katherine. *Everything You Need to Know About Relationship Violence.* New York: Rosen Publishing Group, 2001.

■ DATE RAPE DRUGS

See: Date Rape; Drugs, Alcohol, and Rape

■ DRUG ABUSE AND RAPE

See: Drugs, Alcohol, and Rape; Gang Rape

■ DRUGS, ALCOHOL, AND RAPE

Substance abuse is defined as the abuse of, dependence on, or addiction to alcohol or illicit (illegal) drugs. It has been called the nation's number one health problem. Abuse of drugs and alcohol is a major factor in all forms of violence, including sexual violence and rape. Substance abuse does not cause violence, but it does impair judgment and can result in people doing things they would not otherwise do.

SEXUAL VIOLENCE AND ALCOHOL ABUSE

In many rapes and sexual assaults, the victim, the perpetrator, or both have been drinking. In various research studies, estimates of the prevalence of alcohol use in rapes and other sexual assaults vary widely due to the way drinking is measured, how sexual assault is defined, and which groups are studied. A summary of 18 studies by Roizen in 1997 found that offenders had been drinking in 13–60 percent of incidents. In 2005, researchers reporting from the Department of Justice found that more than 35 percent of rape or sexual assault victims thought that their attacker was under the influence of drugs or alcohol.

A study by Harrington and Leitenberg, conducted in 1994 at four New England colleges, found that nearly all (97 percent) female students who reported a sexual assault by an acquaintance perceived their assailant to be at least "somewhat drunk." In another study in 1996 at an urban college, Abbey found that the assailant had been drinking in 44 percent of sexual assaults against female students. College-age victims are also likely to have been drinking at the time of a sexual assault. In a 2005 study on rape on college campuses, researchers found that almost half of all the attacks were on women who were incapacitated by alcohol or drugs that they had voluntarily consumed. In their New England colleges study, Harrington and Leitenberg reported that 55 percent of all female students who experienced sexual aggression by an acquaintance stated that they themselves were at least "somewhat drunk" at the time. Thirty percent of women at the urban college who had been sexually assaulted were drinking at the time of the assault. That number has remained highly consistent over time.

A 2004 study in the *Journal of Studies on Alcohol* analyzed data compiled from 119 U.S. colleges and universities participating in three Harvard School of Public Health college alcohol surveys over three years. In total, the surveys involved almost 24,000 women. The study found that colleges and universities with higher rates of binge drinking (defined as consuming five or more drinks in a row for men and four or more drinks in a row for women at least once in the past two weeks) also have more rapes. In addition, nearly three-quarters of rape victims reported being intoxicated at the time of the attack.

TEENS SPEAK

While I Was Drunk, Someone Raped Me

I returned to college the week before classes began after spending the summer at home with my family. My girlfriend invited me to a party. I was looking forward to seeing my college friends after the long vacation.

I had a few drinks at the party, but I'm used to drinking and I know how much I can drink and still take care of myself. I was also with a big group of friends, so I felt safe. I had a few beers and then a guy I only know slightly offered me a shot. I don't remember anything else that happened at the party after drinking the shot. When I woke up, it was the next morning, and I was on a couch in a house shared by some of the guys who were at the party. My pants were unzipped and stained. I had bruises on my thighs. I could not remember what had happened, but I knew that I had been raped. I still have no idea who may have done this to me.

In general, studies show that male college students believe that a woman who drinks invites sexual contact or makes it easier for men to initiate such activity. Another study, this one by Fromme and Wendel in 1995, of mostly white, middle-to-upper-middle class fraternity and sorority members, found that the male students believed they were more likely to trick or strong-arm a woman into having sex when they were drunk rather than when sober. A 2007 study performed at a medium-sized southeastern college found that 19 percent of men felt that it would be acceptable to have sex with a woman if her consent was in doubt, but there would be little risk of any serious consequence for them. For example, such an assault would be acceptable if the woman were so drunk that she was incoherent, but the man was pretty sure she wanted to have sex with him and he used a condom to protect her from pregnancy. A large number of men also thought it acceptable, or even expected, to do anything they could to make a woman more willing to have sex—such as intentionally getting her drunk in order to make her easier to convince.

Fact Or Fiction?

Sexual assaults that involve alcohol are no different from attacks that do not involve alcohol.

The Facts: Although there are similarities, assaults that involve drinking are more likely to take place between men and women who do not know each other well (strangers, acquaintances, or casual dates as opposed to steady dates or spouses). They are also more likely to take place at parties or bars than in the home.

SEXUAL VIOLENCE AND ILLICIT DRUG USE

Like alcohol, illicit drugs can lower inhibitions and make it more difficult to recognize risky situations. In addition, some sexual offenders use drugs secretly and deliberately to incapacitate a victim so that he or she can be more easily assaulted.

Club drugs

Club drugs is the term often used to describe a number of illicit drugs that are most commonly encountered at nightclubs and all-night parties called raves. Although many different kinds of drugs are available at clubs and raves, the three primary club drugs are ecstasy, ketamine, and GHB (gamma hydroxybutyrate). Mixing these drugs with alcohol can greatly enhance (increase) their effects and make a potential victim more susceptible to unwanted sexual activity and aggression. They may also make it less likely that the victim will recognize the danger or be able to defend himself or herself.

Predatory drugs

Predatory drugs, a term used by law enforcement to describe drugs that are used by offenders to facilitate a sexual assault, are also sometimes known as "rape drugs." An assailant sometimes slips

DID YOU KNOW?

The Most Underreported Violent Crime in America

In 2005, 38.3 percent of rapes and sexual assaults were reported to the police.

Source: National Crime Victimization Survey, U.S. Department of Justice, Bureau of Justice Statistics, 2006.

predatory drugs into a drink without the victim's knowledge to render the victim unconscious or otherwise unable to resist sexual advances. The most common predatory drugs are Rohypnol, ketamine, and GHB.

Sexual assaults facilitated by predatory drugs can be difficult to prosecute or even recognize for several reasons. The drugs are invisible and odorless when dissolved in water and have only a mild salty taste easily disguised by soda, juice, liquor, or beer. As a result, victims may not be aware that they have ingested a drug at all. Due to memory problems caused by the drugs, the victim may not be aware of an attack until eight to 12 hours after it occurred. Finally, because the drugs are **metabolized** (processed by the body) quickly, the police may be unable to prove that the drugs were used to facilitate an assault, even if the victim has a blood test.

It may be difficult to determine if an individual was drugged without his or her knowledge before being sexually assaulted. Some signs of a victim's having been drugged include:

- Feeling more intoxicated than expected
- Experiencing a memory lapse and being unable to account for a period of time
- Feeling as if one has had sex but with no memory of the incident

Not everyone is affected by these drugs in the same way. The effects may also vary depending upon the drug, the amount consumed, and whether the drug was mixed with alcohol or other drugs. An individual's weight, gender, metabolism, and how soon he or she received medical assistance may also affect the response.

Q & A

Question: I was drinking at a party and fell asleep. A guy I know had sex with me after I fell asleep. Was I raped?

Answer: Having sex with someone who cannot give consent because of the mental or physical effects of alcohol or drugs is considered a rape. Having sex with someone who cannot resist or say "no" because the person is drugged, drunk, "too out of it," passed out, unconscious, or asleep can also be rape.

To protect oneself from predatory drugs, experts suggest the following:

- Don't accept drinks from anyone except trusted friends
- Personally open all bottles and containers
- Never leave a drink unattended
- Don't share drinks
- Don't drink from punch bowls or other large, common, open containers that may have drugs in them
- Don't drink anything that tastes or smells strange.

See also: Abusive Sexual Behavior; Prevention of Rape: Being Proactive; Prevention of Rape: Being Reactive; Rape Kits and Evidence Collection

FURTHER READING

Aretha, David. *On the Rocks: Teens and Alcohol.* Danbury, Conn.: Childrens Press, 2007.

Hyde, Margaret O., and John F. Setaro. *Alcohol 101: An Overview for Teens.* Fairfield, IA: 21st Century Books, 1999.

■ EDUCATING THE COMMUNITY

Educational programs offering general information on the prevention of rape and other sexual assaults are available in many communities. Some programs also focus on how to deal compassionately with victims of sexual assault. Violence prevention can be described on three levels: primary prevention, or prevention of the rape altogether; secondary prevention, where the perpetrator stops being violent or the victim ceases to be victimized; and tertiary prevention, which involves the victim trying to overcome the trauma of the event. The basic premise of most rape education programs maintains that the best way to prevent sexual violence is through awareness.

INCREASING POLICE AWARENESS

The majority of rapes and other sexual assaults are never reported to the police. The reason lies, at least in part, in the way law enforcement has traditionally viewed victims of rape—particularly date rape. In the past, many women who reported being raped by someone they knew were not believed; often they were ridiculed or told that they had "asked for it." Some also believe, rightly or wrongly, that the police are unlikely to arrest the assailant, particularly when he or she is an intimate partner or spouse of the victim. Some groups of victims, including immigrants, prostitutes, lesbians, and teens, are particularly reluctant to involve the police in cases of rape.

Many of these concerns are based on reality. In the past, many police officers lacked knowledge of the realities of rape and sexual assault. Without that knowledge, they could not effectively deal with the victims or their assailants. Because the police are usually a rape victim's first contact with the criminal justice system, the treatment he or she receives from the officer on call may determine whether he or she files a complaint or drops the case. Today, most police departments provide their officers with rape education, awareness programs, and sensitivity training.

Police officers are asked to understand the particular issues victims of sexual assault face. Rape victims are often traumatized by their experience. Officers must be trained to elicit information in a caring, nonjudgmental fashion. Unfortunately, some officers do not realize that a domestic partner or spouse can be guilty of rape. Others know very little about date rape, or drug-facilitated rape. In order for the courts to fully prosecute these crimes, they require that police officers gain sensitivity to the dangers posed by the assailant and to the fears of the victim. Police officers are also taught how to collect and store the evidence of DNA, the genetic information essential to living cells that controls inherited characteristics and sometimes helps identify, and later prosecute, a rapist.

Fact Or Fiction?

Telling the police what happened to me will make me feel worse.

The Facts: Many rape victims actually feel better after talking to the police. Reporting the crime can help you regain a sense of personal power and control. You may feel less victimized as a result. You may also feel like you are helping prevent a similar assault from occurring to someone else.

EFFECTIVE SCHOOL PROGRAMS

Educational programs are designed to teach children and teens how to keep themselves safe from sexual assault. Counselors and educators try to break down the myths surrounding rape and to help counteract the stigma and embarrassment often felt by the victims of sexual assault. The programs vary depending on the age of the students.

For elementary school children, dramatic enactments are common. One such program is "Good Touch, Bad Touch, Secret Touch," which uses puppets named Run and Tell to teach about appropriate touching and rules that can help keep youngsters safe. In general, very young children are taught that their bodies are private and that if anyone touches them inappropriately, they must tell an adult as soon as possible, regardless of what an abuser may have told them.

National hotlines and help sites, such as the National Domestic Hotline or RAINN (Rape, Abuse, & Incest National Network), will refer callers seeking help to local rape crisis centers, many of which have programs to help older students and in which educators can find information and advice. Typically, these programs contain information about the services offered by the center, statistics on rape and sexual assault, explanations of what happens to offenders after their conviction, the long-term emotional and psychological effects of sexual assault on victims and their families, and strategies for preventing rapes.

Peer education programs are another way of educating teens about sexual violence. These programs encourage young people to share what they learn with their peers.

Q & A

Question: When the police did a presentation at my school, they said to tell a trusted adult if we were being abused. Can I tell my teacher and not have her report it to the police?

Answer: Your teacher is required by law to report abuse. That doesn't mean you shouldn't confide in him or her. A teacher may be able to assist you in getting the help you need.

Rape prevention programs usually try to dispel myths about rape as well as include discussions of how to handle various situations. Many college students also place some blame on the sexual assault victim, particularly when alcohol is involved. A 2007 study of beliefs about blame in college students found that both male and female students believed the woman to be more responsible for an attack if she was drunk. Prevention programs try to expose such myths and help change student attitudes about sexual aggression. Some high schools and colleges offer self-defense training programs that may help students reduce the risk of sexual assault. They identify potentially threatening situations and teach students skills that might thwart an attacker.

Several programs at the high school level have been studied to see if they are effective. For example, the Centers for Disease Control and Prevention (CDC) conducted a study in 2000 of eighth and ninth graders in rural North Carolina. A program of school and community activities teaches students primary prevention of dating violence by changing norms associated with partner violence, decreasing gender stereotyping, and improving conflict management skills. Activities encourage secondary prevention by also changing beliefs about the need for help, improving awareness of services for victims and perpetrators, and modeling help-seeking behavior. Those who attended the program were found in follow-up studies to have committed less psychological abuse, less sexual violence, and less violence against the current dating partner.

Another program, the Youth Relationships Program, an 18-week mixed-gender group program designed for at-risk youths ages 14-16, also showed promising results. Compared with a group of at-risk youths who did not receive the program, young people who received the program indicated less use of coercive behavior in their relationships at a six-month follow-up study. Several other studies have evaluated the effectiveness of date rape prevention programs in reducing the incidence of sexual assault. Although most of these programs show an increase in knowledge around risky behaviors and date rape, some have found that women—particularly those who have been victimized in the past—still remain at risk for future victimization. A few studies have even shown negative results in male participants, who may develop a defensive attitude about their beliefs and behavior after having received the information in a rape prevention program.

TEENS SPEAK

I Didn't Want Anyone to Know I Had Been Raped

I got raped. It was horrible, and I didn't want my parents to know. They are older and from a different country and culture. I knew they wouldn't understand.

I thought that if I reported the crime to the police that they would tell my parents. But I didn't want my rapist to get away with what he did to me either. I also didn't want him to get the chance to do to another girl what he did to me.

One day at school a police officer came in to give a presentation to my class. She said that if we were raped we could make a report to the police without telling our parents. I was so relieved.

OTHER GROUPS

A number of other groups in communities across the nation also receive training related to rape and sexual violence. Medical students are taught how to compassionately and effectively treat victims of sexual violence and collect the medical evidence necessary to help convict the assailant. They are also educated to recognize signs of sexual abuse in any children they treat.

Teachers and day-care workers also are expected to be aware of the signs of sexual abuse in their students. They are required by law to report any suspected abuse of children and teens.

Training programs are also available to self-defense instructors, who may encounter victims of assault in their classes; to parents interested in protecting their children from sexual abuse; to people who work with victims of domestic violence; to lawyers, judges, and other legal workers; and to social service workers.

Educational programs are also available to the general population of a community. These programs can help individuals learn how to protect themselves from sexual assault and identify where and how to seek help in the event that they are attacked. Some places to go for help are listed at the back of this book.

See also: Help and Support; Prevention of Rape: Being Proactive; Rape in the Media, Reporting; Rape Kits and Evidence Collection

FURTHER READING

Domitrz, Michael. *May I Kiss You? A Candid Look at Dating, Communication, Respect, & Sexual Assault Awareness.* Greenfield, Wis.: Awareness Publications, 2003.

Ferguson, Robert, and Jeanine Ferguson. *A Guide to Rape Awareness and Prevention: Educating Yourself, Your Family and Those in Need.* Wethersfield, Conn.: Turtle Press, 1994.

Feuereisen, Patti. *Invisible Girls: The Truth About Sexual Abuse—A Book for Teen Girls, Young Women, and Everyone Who Cares About Them.* New York: Seal Press, 2005.

■ FEMALE RIGHTS

The status of women in society. The rights of women are closely linked to their likelihood of experiencing **gender-based violence** or rape. In societies where women are more equal to men, there is less violence against them. Therefore, working to improve the rights and equality of women is a way of working to prevent rape and other forms of gender-based violence.

Female rights encompass a large variety of issues. From voting rights to simple human rights, such as the right to attend school, the status of women in a society is often controlled by both law and custom. With respect to a woman's susceptibility to rape, many of these seemingly unrelated areas often turn out to be factors. Protecting women from sexual assault is not simply a matter of keeping them away from the minority of men who might prey on them. It is important to change how men within a society see women in order to address their overall level of risk. Doing so not only requires education but also often specific changes in the laws that affect female rights.

SEXUAL FREEDOM

Women continue to fight for the right to stand equally with men. Whatever successes women have had in trying to achieve equality of pay, equality of opportunity, or even equality of respect, there are still areas in which women are not treated equally to men. One of these areas is in the domain of sexual freedom.

Although rape shield laws prevent the use of a woman's past sexual history against her during a sexual assault trial, many people still assume that rape is less traumatic for women who have chosen to be sexual with more men. Furthermore, there is the assumption that if a woman has had sex with a man once, she will do it again. Therefore, it can be far more difficult to prosecute and convict rapists in cases where the woman has previously agreed to have sex with her attacker. This is also related to the difficulty in prosecuting, and often-reduced penalties for, marital rape cases. Once a woman has agreed to have sex with a man, many people feel there should be an assumption of consent for all future sexual encounters.

DRESS RESTRICTIONS

Women should have the right to dress as they choose without being told that their clothing has invited a sexual assault. Short skirts and low cut tops are not a request for rape. They are not, to quote many attackers, "asking for it." The idea that a woman's style of dress is an invitation to an attack actually reflects a perception of men as uncontrollable sexual animals. It implies that men are not rational, thinking beings with morals and the ability to make intentional decisions. It suggests that the mere sight of legs or cleavage turns men into creatures of instinct instead of reason. Although this is clearly ridiculous, societies across the globe, and across time, have imposed dress restrictions on women at least in part to control men's sexual desire.

In the Victorian era, showing even an ankle was considered to be risqué. Today, different cultures have different ideas about appropriate clothing for women. Some of these expectations reflect an intention to control male sexuality by removing the temptation of the female form, whereas others reflect a perception of women as the property of their fathers or husbands and, therefore, as an asset that needs to be protected.

Certain religious sects require women to dress in particular ways to preserve their modesty. For example, the Christian Church of Jesus Christ of Latter-day Saints, more commonly known as the Mormon church, asks women not to wear revealing clothing, including short shorts and tight pants. Some Catholic churches in Italy also require women to cover their shoulders and knees before they will be allowed to enter. These requirements of modesty are drawn from biblical passages that also determine the modest clothing choices of highly orthodox Jewish women.

Many religious Muslim women also follow specific rules when it comes to their mode of dress. Their attire may range from a simple head covering to a garment that covers them completely from head to toe, including a mesh veil over their eyes. By and large, the coverings are culturally mandated rather than religiously imposed. There is actually more discussion of men's clothing than women's in the Koran. What text there is on women's dress seems largely aimed at protecting women, helping them preserve their autonomy, and allowing them to travel through the world safe from harassment. In more recent times, however, dress restrictions have often been used to restrict women's freedom of movement. That having been said, there is a growing movement in which young Muslim women are choosing the veil as an instrument of female empowerment. They say that hiding their faces, hair, or bodies allows them to exist on an equal footing with men where, otherwise, they would be judged based on superficial characteristics such as their appearance.

Orthodox Jewish women also follow varying levels of dress restriction depending on their culture and particular beliefs. One of the most common things that married Orthodox Jewish women are required to do is cover their hair. This requirement is imposed because hair is considered sensuous; it is thought that a married woman should reserve that side of herself for her husband alone. Observant Orthodox

Jewish women are also often required to keep their shoulders covered, to wear tops that do not show any cleavage, and to dress in skirts or dresses long enough to cover their knees when seated. Pants are often avoided by these women as seemingly less modest, except for women who work in areas where pants are more practical for maintaining modesty during movement.

Although many religious restrictions were initially developed for the seemingly innocuous purposes of preserving a woman's beauty for her husband alone, and keeping women from drawing attention to themselves, in recent years they have taken on a somewhat more disturbing note. Why, after all, many modern women feel, should it be necessary for a woman to cover herself to be safe from men?

SEX SEGREGATION IN ISRAEL

In 2007, there was an incident on a sex-segregated Israeli bus line where an Orthodox Jewish woman refused to move to the back of a bus that was informally designated as sex-segregated. She was badly beaten because of her refusal, and, in the commentary following the event, many individuals, both men and women, in the religious Orthodox community said that the restrictions were in place because men should not be expected to have to control themselves while looking at inappropriately dressed women, or even at any women at all. On sex-segregated buses, women are required to sit in the back so that men do not have to look at them and risk temptation.

Because of this and other similar events, several women filed lawsuits against the Israeli government asking for the sex-segregated buses to be declared illegal. The buses are often the only form of public transportation between various places, and the women believe the sex segregation is fundamentally discriminatory. Even where women would choose to ride the buses, many have been refused entry to a bus or thrown off because of immodest attire. Modesty patrols have also become an issue in certain areas of Israel where ultra-orthodox Haredi men have thrown bleach on women whose attire they found inappropriate.

Some ultra-orthodox women say that it is the removal of the sex-segregated buses that would be discriminatory. As with the Muslim women who find wearing the veil to be a positive experience, these women find it empowering to be able to maintain the sex segregation on which their religion places such a high value—even though the Israeli women described represent a minority of the female population, and Muslim women wearing a veil or head covering in the Middle East are in the majority. They find it gives them strength not to have to be viewed by strange men. Still, social structures that encourage violence against women seem, to many, to be fundamentally flawed, even if they are what some women prefer.

TAKE BACK THE NIGHT

Take Back the Night rallies have become a common sight on many college campuses and some city streets. Although they differ in form from event to event, the goal of every Take Back the Night event is to reduce the amount of violence against women. Take Back the Night rallies are designed to do exactly what their name implies—take back the night so that women can feel like they are safe from sexual violence. These events bring men and women together to promote awareness of sexual violence and educate the population at large as to how the streets can be made safer and sexual assaults can be avoided.

It is widely reported that the Take Back the Night movement started in Europe in the 1970s. However, there is little scholarship to support the claim. There are clear reports of a Take Back the Night march of more than 5,000 women who took to the streets following a 1978 anti-pornography conference in San Francisco, California, but the earliest history of the movement remains unclear. Regardless of the movement's origins, Take Back the Night rallies grew over time from gatherings of feminist women to gatherings of all people, both male and female, who wanted to work to make the streets, and their friends, safe.

Unfortunately, in the early 1990s, there was a decline in attendance at Take Back the Night events because of the scientifically unsupported rape-hype movement. The leaders of the rape-hype movement claimed that acquaintance rape was not really a social problem, and the publicity that grew around their statements reduced support for antiviolence activities. Fortunately, the movement also inspired a great deal of research as to the true prevalence of acquaintance rape and other crimes of sexual violence. As scientists have shown acquaintance rape to be a serious problem, they have re-inspired both women and men to take back the night.

THE VAGINA MONOLOGUES

The Vagina Monologues is an evolving theatrical piece that was the idea of activist, playwright, and actress Eve Ensler. The original play, which has been performed across the United States and around the world, was based on a series of interviews that Ms. Ensler conducted with more than 200 women. The monologues describe real women's experiences with their bodies, ranging from brutal rape to times of extraordinary pleasure. Because of the nature of its subject matter, in the years following its first performance, *The Vagina Monologues* spawned a great deal of controversy. It also inspired a new generation of antiviolence advocates to create the holiday known as V-Day.

V-Day was first celebrated in 1998 and has continued to be celebrated every year since. The goal of V-Day celebrations is to increase awareness of the ongoing problem of violence against women. V-Day celebrations usually include productions of *The Vagina Monologues,* often performed by local celebrities, as well as other awareness-raising events. They have been used to raise money for women's shelters around the world, and the nonprofit foundation that helps produce the events continues to fund various antiviolence organizations across the globe.

FEMALE GENITAL MUTILATION

Female genital mutilation, also known as female circumcision, is practiced in many societies around the world. Female genital mutilation is performed as a range of procedures, from the removal of the **clitoral hood** to infibulation. Infibulation is the amputation of the **clitoris** and clitoral hood, the removal of the **labia majora** and **labia minora**, and then the sewing together of the remaining tissue to leave only a hole big enough for urine and menstrual blood to escape. In general, female genital mutilation is not performed by a physician, and the women it is performed on are at risk of infection as well as other serious complications.

Why do societies perform female genital mutilation? They do it to control female sexuality. It is thought that by removing the parts of the body that allow women to experience pleasure during sexual encounters, the women will remain virgins until marriage and then remain faithful to their husbands. Female genital mutilation may not be rape, but it has some of the same consequences, both mental and physical. The World Health Organization (WHO) has been calling for an end to the practice for decades, as has the United Nations (UN), as part of its Declaration on the Elimination of Violence Against Women.

Unfortunately, female genital mutilation is often so deeply rooted in local culture that it can be difficult to eliminate. In Egypt, for example, a 2008 study found that almost 85 percent of 10-to-14-year-old girls had been circumcised in the six years following the passage of a law forbidding the practice.

HONOR KILLINGS

In some societies, when a woman is raped by a man she is put to death by her family. Why? Because she is considered to have dishonored them by having sex with a man who is not her husband, even though doing so was not her choice. Honor crimes may be loosely defined as violent attacks upon a woman who has disgraced her family by participating in unapproved sexual conduct. Whether a woman was raped, had an affair, or merely engaged in **consensual** sexual intercourse may not matter to her family or a court. The punishment for a woman dishonoring her family in such a way can range from beatings to death.

In many countries, men who kill their sisters, wives, or daughters as part of an honor crime may be eligible for reduced penalties or even full dismissal of the case. A 1996 study of honor killings in Jordan found that 23 of the 38 female homicides in the previous year were honor killings. Of the 16 cases where there were files available for review, reasons for the murders ranged from pregnancy outside of marriage to adultery to simply having a strange man present in the house. Most of the murderers were the women's brothers, although fathers, ex-husbands, and uncles also committed several of the crimes. In the vast majority of cases, the offenders received either no prison sentence at all or only minimal time in jail.

Honor crimes are a problem throughout much of the world. The UN report "The State of the World Population 2000" estimated that as many as 5,000 women are murdered in crimes of honor each year by members of their families. In 2006, one newspaper report found that there were more than 1,200 honor killings of women in Pakistan alone. Honor crimes are not limited to Muslim countries, although they are most common there. Honor killings have been reported in countries as diverse as India, Sweden, and the United Kingdom.

See also: Law and Rape, The; Prevention of Rape: Being Proactive; Rape in the Media, Reporting

FURTHER READING

United Nations Population Fund. "The State of the World Population 2000. Lives Together, Worlds Apart: Men and Women in a Time of Change." New York: The Fund; 2000. Available online. URL: http://www.unfpa.org/swp/2000/english/.

■ GANG RAPE

Gang rape is the sexual assault of a victim in rapid succession by several attackers in a group of usually young people who often band together for criminal purposes. Gang rape is also known as "group rape" or "party rape." The term *party rape* is often used by college students to refer to gang rapes that occur at parties and other social events.

A single episode of gang rape can include one form of sexual contact (oral rape, for example) or many sexual acts. Victims of gang rape may be raped with objects, such as bottles or hoses. Gang rape is a crime, and anyone who participates in the assault may be prosecuted, including those who watched but did not take part in the rape.

Gang rape occurs less frequently than a sexual assault by a single offender. Statistics from the Department of Justice in 2005 indicated that approximately 18 percent of rapes and sexual assaults are committed by multiple offenders. This is consistent with a 1997 survey by the Commonwealth Fund on the health of adolescent girls that found that multiple perpetrators were responsible for 16 percent of completed rapes and 10 percent of attempted rapes. A gang rape can occur anywhere but is more common on college campuses and in areas where large numbers of young people gather. The most frequent perpetrators of gang rapes are young men and teenage boys.

Fact Or Fiction?

Only men commit gang rape, and the only victims are women.

The Facts: Gangs of teenagers—young women as well as young men—have committed gang rapes. Men and boys are also victims of gang rape. These attacks are usually perpetrated by men and boys who consider themselves heterosexual.

CHARACTERISTICS OF PARTICIPANTS IN A GANG RAPE

Although every gang rape is unique, gang rapes as a whole tend to share some characteristics. First, the individuals who commit the rape usually know each other and share a group identity. Members of the group tend to share values and beliefs; they may be members of a sports team or belong to a teenage gang.

Most individuals who participate in a gang rape are aggressive (both physically and sexually), competitive, and intensely loyal to the other members of their group. They also tend to view women as sex objects rather than equals. Most have hostile attitudes toward women and tend to believe that the women they rape "wanted it." They often comment that a woman who has had more than two drinks or is dressed in revealing clothing is advertising that she wants sex. They wrongly believe that these two behaviors make gang rape acceptable.

Q & A

Question: Are boys and men who gang rape so oversexed that they can't control themselves?

Answer: According to health science journalist Robin Warshaw, author of *I Never Called It Rape*, gang rapes are not about sexual desire or a need for sexual fulfillment. Men and boys who commit gang rapes are under enormous peer pressure to prove their strength and manhood to their group. By participating, they believe they are proving that they are "real men." They also think that taking part in a gang rape is a bonding experience, one that shows that their group is dominant, powerful, and superior (over other men and all women).

GANG RAPE ON COLLEGE CAMPUSES

Gang rape is not an uncommon occurrence at many colleges and universities, particularly at those on which social life revolves around fraternities and college team sports. According to sociologists Carol Bohmer and Andrea Parrot, authors of *Sexual Assault on Campus: The Problem and the Solution* (1993), in their research sample, fraternity members committed 55 percent of the alleged gang rapes and athletes were responsible for 40 percent. At Brigham Young University there were two separate incidents where football players were accused of gang rape in 2004 alone. Gang rapes have also been associated with men who live in the same residence hall, but these rapes are less common.

An important characteristic of gang rapes on college campuses is that both the assailants and their victims have usually consumed large quantities of alcohol or drugs. In fact, college groups that engage in gang rape, such as some fraternities and athletic teams, tend to promote drinking as a way to relax, have fun, or socialize. Members of these groups are expected to consume large quantities of alcohol. If a potential member does not participate, he is usually rejected for membership.

Psychologists and sociologists who have studied gang rape on college campuses emphasize that the heavy alcohol use makes out-of-control sexual behavior more likely, just as alcohol abuse increases the possibilities of other forms of rape.

College students who commit gang rape typically try to get their victims intoxicated so that they will be ready for sex. At parties, for example, beer and hard liquor are often the only beverages available. Sometimes the only drink served is an alcohol-spiked punch. In addition, drinking games are a frequent source of entertainment.

TEENS SPEAK

My Friend Is Innocent, But His Teammates Raped a Girl

My friend is in trouble with the law because some guys on his hockey team supposedly gang-raped a girl at a victory party after the championship game. At first he said he had nothing to do with the rape; he was just in the room when it happened, but the police think he was involved.

A few weeks ago, he told me that when the guys started to gang up on the girl, he knew what was going to happen but felt powerless to stop it. The toughest and most popular boys were the ringleaders, and he felt that if he said anything, they would call him a wimp and never let him hang out with them again. He didn't join them, but he watched it happen, partly because he knew that was what they expected.

He says that ever since that night, he can't get the cries of the girl or the cheers of the boys off his mind. He wishes more than anything that he could just go back in time and live that night all over again. He believes he couldn't make them stop raping her, but he could have warned her when they started ganging up on her, and he could have called the police.

PREVENTING GANG RAPE

Of all types of rape, gang rapes are the ones most likely to make headlines. The media tends to sensationalize cases because many people regard it as a baffling and horrifying crime. What the newspapers leave out, however, is a discussion of what motivates a group of teens or college students to commit a gang rape. The media also does not usually reveal what educators and other experts are doing to prevent these crimes.

Many groups on college campuses are working to end gang rape. College administrators have established rules for parties given by fraternities and athletic teams. Some ban alcohol at all social events. Others call on campus police to routinely check parties. A few have abolished fraternities in an attempt to encourage social events that are not solely based on alcohol or drug use.

A number of colleges and universities are taking a different approach. They are educating students, both men and women, about rape on campus. It is becoming more common for members of male athletic teams to participate in sexual assault awareness programs. These classes use facts to undermine common myths about rape, such as, "Women who say no to sex really mean that they want it." These programs also try to broaden athletes' understanding by introducing athletes to women's views about rape and the experiences of rape victims. At some colleges, all incoming first-year students must take part in a rape prevention program.

A number of psychologists and sociologists are gathering information about gang rapes to better understand how these assaults can be prevented. They view their studies of groups who are prone to these crimes as key to developing improved methods of prevention. According to sociologist Patricia Yancey Martin, however, much more work still needs to be done.

PROTECTION FROM GANG RAPE?

Protecting oneself from gang rape is, in many ways, no different from protecting oneself from other forms of rape. Because alcohol is commonly involved in episodes of gang rape, avoiding alcohol and drugs at parties and other social events is an important strategy.

Experts suggest that teens attend parties with friends who agree to look out for one another. Before arriving at a party, a teen should have a plan for getting home safely. In creating that plan, young people should steer clear of groups loitering on the sidewalks, in parking lots, in alleys, and in front of stores. If anyone blocks access to one's car or home, he or she should return to a safe area where there are other people. If these groups do not allow you to leave, call the police.

Many counselors encourage teens to attend rape prevention programs at their school or in their community. By educating themselves and participating in efforts to make their environment a safer place, they are sending the signal that they care about having a safe community to live in, that they believe in putting an end to rape, and that they are not going to be the type of person that looks the other way as far as rape is concerned.

See also: Date Rape; Drugs, Alcohol, and Rape; Male Role in Rape; Prevention of Rape: Being Proactive; Prevention of Rape: Being Reactive; Rape in the Media, Reporting; Sexual Assault, Types of

FURTHER READING

Miller, Jody. *Getting Played: African American Girls, Urban Inequality, and Gendered Violence.* New York: New York University Press, 2008.

Sanday, Peggy. *Fraternity Gang Rape.* New York: New York University Press, 2007.

■ HELP AND SUPPORT

Victims need support, not only from family members and friends, but also from law enforcement and medical personnel. Victims usually also require the services of professionals to overcome some of the long-term psychological effects of rape.

SUPPORT GROUPS

Most communities and many college campuses have rape crisis centers. These centers are largely staffed by volunteers (many of whom have also experienced sexual assault), and the centers usually provide a variety of services, such as hotline crisis counseling, adolescent and family services, support groups, medical advocacy, and legal advocacy. Many also offer education on issues related to sexual violence to schools, community groups, teen centers, and businesses. Frequently, the services offered by rape crisis centers are free or low cost.

Many college campuses also have rape crisis centers that offer some of the same services as community-based centers. Even on campuses where there is no designated crisis center, counseling staff may be available to assist victims of sexual assault. The staff provides support services for students who have been sexually assaulted, including help in finding medical, police, legal, and counseling assistance. Many also offer assistance in changing class schedules and living arrangements when necessary.

Anyone who has been raped on a college campus may need to report the crime to the campus security force as well as the local police department. If the assailant is a student, he or she will most likely face disciplinary proceedings at school in addition to legal proceedings in criminal court.

Many colleges offer educational programs related to rape prevention, particularly during freshman orientation. Education concerning date rape can be especially important on college campuses. Escort services, where campus police transport women and men who would otherwise need to walk alone at night, are also sometimes available.

LAW ENFORCEMENT

Reporting a rape to law enforcement authorities can be emotionally difficult. However, only if a victim reports the rape can the perpetrator be brought to justice and punished. Yet many victims of sexual assault find that reporting the crime gives them a sense of control and empowerment. Most prefer to take a friend or family member with them when they report a sexual assault, as telling strangers about the experience can be painful.

Fact Or Fiction?

All sexual assault victims report the crime immediately to the police. If they do not report it or delay in reporting it, then they must have changed their minds after it happened, wanted revenge, or didn't want to look like they were sexually active.

The Facts: There are many reasons why victims may not report a rape to the police. A delay in reporting does *not* mean that the victim thinks the offender should get away with his crime. It is not easy to talk about being sexually assaulted. The experience of telling what happened may cause the person to relive the trauma. The victims may fear retaliation by the offender, that they won't be believed, that they will be blamed for the assault, or that the offender will not be held accountable even if they tell. Some want to just forget the assault ever happened, while others feel shame or shock.

Although law enforcement personnel should help victims through the various steps of the legal process, many are too busy or lack sensitivity to the needs of rape victims. Therefore, many victims look elsewhere for support in negotiating the legal system.

In some communities, victims turn to advocacy groups that assist individuals who are fearful of testifying or facing their assailant in court. Their help may also include someone to talk to in confidence, a pre-trial visit to the courtroom to look around before being called as a witness, information on court procedures, a quiet place to wait before and during the hearing, and someone to accompany the victim into the courtroom. Many advocacy groups also provide practical help with expense forms, specific answers to questions about the case, and a chance to discuss the case when it has ended and receive more help and information.

SUPPORT FOR CHILDREN

When a child has been sexually abused, the reactions of parents and other family members can play an important role in protecting him or her. The family should neither minimize the abuse nor overreact to the situation.

Most experts warn against criticizing or blaming the child for the abuse. They believe it is necessary that the child understand that he or she has done nothing wrong. The abuse is the fault of the offender, not the child. Experts also encourage family members to respect the child's privacy and support him or her in the decision to tell others about what happened.

Q & A

Question: Can a child who was sexually abused ever recover from the experience?

Answer: In many cases, children do recover. Most children are amazingly resilient. Research suggests that children who receive support when their abuse becomes known heal more quickly than those who are not believed. A supportive family and professional intervention and counseling can also help to heal child victims and their families.

DID YOU KNOW?

Sex of Victims and Perpetrators of Rape

According to the Department of Justice, in 96 percent of reported date rapes, males were the perpetrators and females were the victims. In about 2 percent of all cases, both the perpetrators and the victims were male, and in 1 percent of all cases, females were the perpetrators and males the victims; in the final 1 percent, both the perpetrators and victims were female.

Children who are victims of rape should receive appropriate medical care, and law enforcement should be notified. The family may also wish to alert a child protection agency or other social services organizations that work in cooperation with law enforcement. The need for counseling or therapy for the child and the entire family should be considered. For help, or to report a child who is being abused, contact the National Center for Missing and Exploited Children. See the Hotlines and Help Sites section at the back of this book to contact the center and to find other sources of support.

SUPPORT FOR PARENTS OF
SEXUALLY ABUSED CHILDREN

Parents of children who have been sexually abused often need professional assistance or support from other parents in learning to cope with the attack. In addition to learning how to support and help their child, the parents may need support themselves. They may blame themselves for not being able to protect the youngster or may feel that they are not good parents. Support groups within the community or on the Internet may help parents to connect with others who have undergone a similar experience. Counseling, both individual and family therapy, can also be helpful.

WHAT TO DO IF RAPE OCCURS

If you or someone you know has been raped, the first thing to do is to reach a safe place and call a family member or a friend for support. Those who wish to report the crime should notify the police immediately.

Initial steps

All physical evidence of the assault should be preserved. The victim should not shower or bathe until he or she has had a medical examination. Every article of clothing worn at the time of the assault should be placed in separate paper (not plastic) bags. It is also important not to clean or disturb the area where the assault occurred. The victim should try to record as much as he or she can remember about the circumstances of the assault, including a description of the assailant. To answer questions about how best to report the crime, receive medical care, or tell friends or family what happened, victims should call a rape crisis center, a hotline, or other victim assistance agencies.

Getting medical help

As soon as possible after the assault, the victim should go to a hospital emergency room or a specialized clinic that provides treatment for victims of sexual assault. Even if the victim believes he or she has no physical injuries, he or she should still be examined for sexually transmitted diseases. Female victims should also discuss with a health-care provider the possibility of pregnancy. Having a medical exam is also a way to preserve physical evidence of a sexual assault. The doctor will use a rape kit to collect fibers, hairs, saliva, semen, and other evidence that the attacker may have left behind. If the victim suspects that he or she may have been given a rape drug, he or she should ask the hospital or clinic to take a urine sample. Drugs such as Rohypnol and GHB are more likely to be detected in urine than in blood.

Reporting rape

If the victim decides to report a rape, he or she should do so immediately. Reporting the crime can help the victim regain a sense of personal power and control. If the assailant is caught and convicted, it also ensures that he cannot do the same thing to someone else.

The importance of talking and counseling

Counseling can help victims learn how to cope with the emotional and physical impacts of the assault. While most people may just want to put the incident behind him or her, talking about it with a counselor who is trained to assist rape victims often helps them heal faster. To find a counselor, contact a local rape crisis center, a hotline, a counseling service, other victim assistance agencies, or RAINN (Rape, Abuse & Incest National Network; (800) 656-HOPE). RAINN is a national victim assistance organization that connects victims to a rape crisis center in their area.

TEENS SPEAK

I Was Raped Three Years Ago
When I Was Fifteen

When it happened, the rapist told me not to tell anyone and I didn't. No one knew, not even my mom or my best friend.

Even though I never saw the rapist again, I felt he still had power over me. The secret was eating me up.

About a year ago, I finally got into counseling and started talking to my close friends about what happened. Last week, I went to the police. I thought they would be unwilling to help me because it had been so long since the attack, but they were very professional about it. They took my report and told me they would try and find the rapist. Even if they never do find him, I feel stronger because I reported him. I was silent then, but I'm not silent now.

IF A FRIEND IS RAPED

If someone you know is raped, he or she will need you to be there for him or her. The support and understanding of friends and family members can help a sexual assault victim heal much faster. Let your friend know that you care and want to help.

Your friend may or may not want to talk about the assault. Let your friend decide when to talk about the attack. Do not press for details or ask a lot of questions. Make sure your friend knows you believe him or her. Many victims remain silent because they feel ashamed or fear that they will not be believed or will even be blamed if they tell other people.

Although it is up to your friend to notify police or contact a rape crisis center, do what you can to assist him or her in getting information about these and other options. Encourage your friend to get medical care, even if the assault happened some time ago and even if your friend does not appear to have any physical injuries. You should also encourage your friend to talk with a counselor at a rape treatment center. If at all possible, offer to accompany your friend to get help.

See also: Educating the Community; Prevention of Rape: Being Reactive; Rape Kits and Evidence Collection; Safe Areas, Establishing

FURTHER READING
Atkinson, Matt. *Resurrection After Rape: A Guide to Transforming from Victim to Survivor.* Oklahoma City, Oklahoma: R.A.R. Publishing, 2008.
Ledray, Linda E. *Recovering from Rape.* New York: Owl Books, 1994.

■ INTERNET PREDATORS

Individuals who use the Internet to take advantage of vulnerable people, usually sexually or financially. While some Internet predators only engage in online sexual activities with their prey, others also use the Internet to lure victims offline.

According to the U.S. Census Bureau, 60 to 80 percent of young people between the ages of 10 and 17 had access to the Internet in 2003. That number is even higher today, as Internet-enabled devices become more widely available both in schools and at home. While the Internet is a wonderful tool, it does have its hazards. The Center for Missing and Exploited Children (CMEC) has calculated that Internet victimization affects the lives of hundreds of thousands, if not millions, of young people each year.

SEXUAL ABUSE ON THE INTERNET

Many types of sexual abuse can occur online. In 2005, the CMEC found that 13 percent of the 10-to-17-year-olds using the Internet were solicited for sex online, and 4 percent were approached in a way that they found aggressive or distressing. Even greater numbers of young people were exposed to sexual images they did not wish to view or were otherwise sexually harassed.

Unwanted exposure to sexual images

More than one-third of Internet-using teens have been exposed to sexual images they did not want to see. The CMEC found that almost one out of every 10 teens has viewed images that he or she found not only unpleasant but disturbing. Most of these exposures are not the result of specific attacks. Instead, large numbers of teenagers come across sexual images while searching for legitimate information on the Internet. Many pornographic Web sites take advantage of misspellings of common search terms in order to lure individuals to their sites, and once on such a site it can be very hard to find a way to leave. More problematic are individuals who approach teens and intentionally send them sexual images and videos. **Exhibitionism** is a major component of online sex crimes, and many predators send explicit photographs of themselves to their victims.

Requests for sexual information and photos

Often, Internet predators will engage their victims in conversations about sex. No one should ever feel obligated to talk about sex or

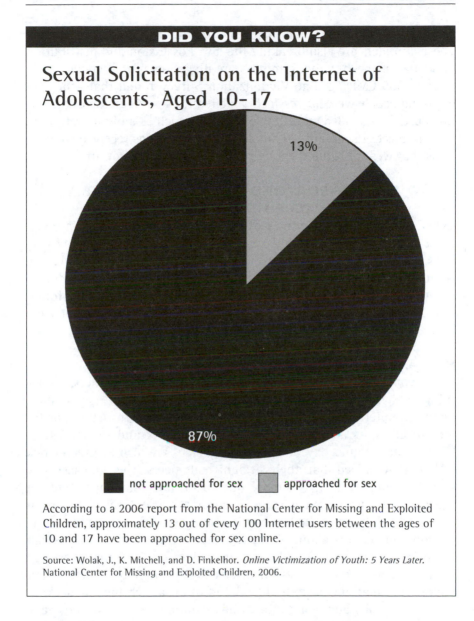

DID YOU KNOW?

Sexual Solicitation on the Internet of Adolescents, Aged 10–17

13%

87%

■ not approached for sex   ▨ approached for sex

According to a 2006 report from the National Center for Missing and Exploited Children, approximately 13 out of every 100 Internet users between the ages of 10 and 17 have been approached for sex online.

Source: Wolak, J., K. Mitchell, and D. Finkelhor. *Online Victimization of Youth: 5 Years Later.* National Center for Missing and Exploited Children, 2006.

reveal sexual information about himself or herself to strangers. It is none of their business, and it can be a prelude to other forms of sexual solicitation, including requests for revealing or sexually explicit photos. Such photos are always a bad idea to take. Even if a teen feels like he or she has developed a **consensual,** trusting relationship with the person requesting them, that person is taking advantage of the teen. These strangers are also breaking the law. Possession and distribution of sexual images involving minors are illegal acts in all states.

The 2005 CMEC Online Victimization Survey found that 4 percent of young people were *aggressively* solicited for sex. Aggressive solicitations usually included an offline component such as a phone call or an offer to meet or send gifts. A similar number of teens received solicitations that were disturbing enough to make them upset or afraid.

HOW PREDATORS USE THE INTERNET TO FIND VICTIMS

Cyber crimes are often crimes of opportunity, but not always. Even those predators who take advantage of a situation, instead of targeting a specific individual, often have a type of victim they seek. The National Juvenile Online Victimization (NJOV) study of law-enforcement agencies, which looked at sex crimes on the Internet, found that 75 percent of victims were young women and 76 percent were between 13 and 15 years old.

How are victims chosen?

Some young people are more appealing victims than others, something which has nothing to do with their physical appearance. Regularly interacting with strangers online is a known risk factor for victimization, as is specifically talking about sex and sexual issues. Women, and young gay or questioning men, are also at greater risk of being victimized than their straight male peers. The increased risk seen in young women is simply due to the fact that most Internet predators are heterosexual men. In contrast, young gay men are at increased risk because the Internet is often their only source for information and support about issues relating to their sexuality. This can leave them open to manipulation by predators who initially present themselves as safe resources for discussing sensitive questions. Other factors that may increase the likelihood of an attack include seeking out pornography and being rude or nasty online. These activities have been shown to draw the attention of Internet predators.

Who are sexual predators?

Most online sexual predators are adult men. It is very easy for adults to access teens on the Internet. In the Pew Internet study of teenage life online, more than half of teens using the Internet had exchanged instant messages with a stranger, and most of them did not see doing so as a problem.

Not all sexual predators, however, are people one might suspect. The CMEC survey found that, stunningly, 14 percent of unwanted sexual solicitations and 44 percent of harassments were by individuals who young people knew offline. Furthermore, sexual harassment and solicitation do not only occur in the privacy of a teenager's room. Approximately one-third of all incidents occurred when teens were on the Internet in the company of their friends.

Chat rooms

Predators will often spend time sitting in chat rooms waiting for an appropriate victim. After monitoring the conversation, predators have been known to use the information they have gathered to try and lure their target into a private chat. Eventually, these predators may attempt to convince their victim to meet them in person. Fortunately, as Internet safety education improves, fewer and fewer young adults are using chat rooms to talk to strangers, and the number of chat room solicitations has declined. Still, the NJOV study found that 76 percent of Internet-initiated sex crimes began with contact in a chat room.

Social networking sites

Social networking sites are incredibly popular among teenagers. A Pew research study estimated that more than half of all teen Internet users have profiles on one or more sites. Disturbingly, despite the fact that most teens are using social networking sites to stay connected to people they already know, only 66 percent limit views of their profiles to their current friends. This means that all the personal details of their lives, including photos and plans, may be available to anyone using the Internet.

Exploiting weakness

Encouraging teenagers to run away from home is a popular tactic of Internet predators. Anyone who encourages a teen to run away from home should be treated with a great deal of suspicion. If a teen does not feel safe at home, there are organizations, such as the National Runaway Switchboard (1-800-RUNAWAY), that can help him or her get out. An individual on the Internet who offers to help a teen run away may actually be trying to lure him or her into greater danger.

Many predators also use gifts as a way to entice their young victims to reveal information about themselves or to meet them in person. The NJOV study found that almost half of all Internet sex crimes involved the perpetrators offering or sending their prey money or gifts. This is a very effective ploy, as The Internet and The Family 2000 study found that 40 percent of teens were willing to give out their personal information in exchange for the offer of a gift worth $100 or more.

Statutory rape

Many Internet predators do not lie to their victims about their age or their interest in sex. Instead, they entice young people with promises of romance and relationships, and most victims of online sex crimes go willingly to their sexual encounters. In fact, in the NJOV study, 73 percent of youth who had sexual encounters with a predator did so more than once. These are crimes of manipulation, not crimes of violence. About 95 percent of Internet-initiated sex crime arrests were for incidents that did not involve force.

Statutory rape laws were created precisely for cases like these. Statutory rape is defined as sex where one of the participants is below the legal age of consent, an age that varies from state to state. Any person who has sex with someone who is below the legal age of consent can be found guilty of statutory rape whether the person's partner said yes or not.

KEEPING SAFE ON THE INTERNET

On the Internet, everything lasts forever. Information that you put online is saved by computers all over the globe, and there is no good way to get rid of it. Therefore, it is important to think very carefully before posting information about yourself on the Internet. Once it is out there, you can never really take it back.

Do not share personal information

Teens should never post personally identifying information on the Internet. Keeping their name, age, location, Social Security number, and credit card information private can help prevent potential predators from locating them and taking advantage of them. Even information that provides only indirect clues to a person's identity can cause problems when posted on public sites.

Fact Or Fiction?

I don't use my real name on my social-networking profile; therefore, no one can tell who I am.

The Facts: Using a pseudonym is not always sufficient to protect your privacy. Details about where you live, where you shop, and even the name of your school's mascot can provide clues to your identity that a predator can use to find you offline. If you don't want people to know who you are, it is important to be very careful about what details about your life you reveal. It's also important to choose a pseudonym that doesn't say too much about you. You shouldn't, for example, pick a user name that includes your real name, age, location, or birth date.

Photographs

A teen who sends an innocent photo to the wrong person, might, in a few days, find naked pictures with his or her face on them spread all over the Internet. It is easy for someone to manipulate digital images to put one person's head on another person's body. It is also important to remember that images from a Web cam can easily be captured, saved, and shared, and that even friends might not respect others' privacy. No one should do anything on a Web cam that they would not be comfortable with their friends seeing the next day at school. In general, a good guideline is that if a person would not want his or her mom, dad, or other adult caregiver to see a picture, it should not be posted on the Internet.

Reporting abuse and harassment

If someone is the victim of harassment on the Internet, it is important that he or she report it to the proper authorities. Some guidelines for what should be reported include requests for personal information from strangers, threatening or harassing e-mails, messages that contain or ask for sexual photos or information, and sites that use trickery to lure people into viewing pornography. In general, any communication on the Internet that makes you uncomfortable should be reported to a parent or teacher; there are also Web sites that can be used to report inappropriate or frightening activities.

Q & A

Question: Someone has been harassing me on the Internet. I told my parents about it, and they called the police. Is there anything else I should do?

Answer: The **CyberTipline** (www.cybertipline.com) is run by the Center for Missing and Exploited Children and should be used to report any sexual exploitation of a minor online or offline, from sexual solicitations to e-mails containing explicit photos that were sent without a request to Web sites that seem legitimate but actually contain pornography. Other useful Web sites include **I-Safe** (www.i-safe.org) and **Wired Safety** (www.wiredsafety.org). I-Safe is a congressionally endorsed nonprofit organization dedicated to educating youth about online safety, and Wired Safety also provides a wide range of information to help you protect yourself on the Internet.

IF YOU DO CHOOSE TO MEET SOMEONE FROM THE INTERNET

Not everyone on the Internet is a predator. Sometimes the cool kid you have been chatting with is exactly who he or she seems to be. However, until you actually meet the electronic correspondent face-to-face, there is no way to be sure. If there is someone with whom you have been talking online whom you wish to meet in person, it is very important to do so safely.

Meet in a public, busy place

The first time a person meets someone they know previously only online, he or she should not meet that person alone. A parent might go on the outing, or the person might go out with a group of friends.

Make certain someone knows where you are

Anytime people go out with others that they do not know well, they should tell their parents, teachers, or even their best friends whom they are meeting and where and when they are meeting them. It is also important to let friends or family know when they expect to be home, to call when they first meet up, and then call again when they get back home safely.

Always meet in a public place
The first few times a person meets someone they've known only from the Internet, it should be in a public place. Meeting in a restaurant or coffee shop where many other people are gathered will help protect the person from someone forcing him or her to do something unwanted.

FURTHER READING
Turow, J., and L. Nir. *The Internet and the Family 2000: The View from Parents, the View from Kids.* Philadelphia: University of Pennsylvania, Annenberg Public Policy Center, 2000.
Wolak J., Mitchell K., and D. Finkelhor. *Online Victimization of Youth: 5 Years Later.* Washington, D.C.: National Center for Missing & Exploited Children, 2006.

◼ LAW AND RAPE, THE
The crime of rape is usually tried at the state level, and punishment may differ from state to state. Traditionally, rape and sexual assault laws referred to female victims and male perpetrators. In recent years, however, most states have changed their laws to be gender neutral.

HISTORY OF RAPE LAWS
Oddly enough, the words *rape*, *rapture*, and *raptor* all come from the same source, the Latin word meaning "to seize." The word *raptor* refers to predatory animals, and *rapture* has a spiritual or romantic meaning. Originally, however, the word *rapture* referred to the act of abducting a virgin for the purpose of marriage. *Rape* also once meant to "take away." Poetry and paintings of the past use the word *rape* where people today use the words *theft* or *kidnapping*.

Until the 1970s, rape laws in the United States were based on the English Common Law, the legal tradition that became the foundation of

America's legal system. English Common Law is more than 700 years old. It developed at a time when the position of women was quite different from what it is today. Hundreds of years ago, English judges treated rape as a property crime. A wife belonged to her father and later her husband, and rape essentially damaged a man's property.

As laws on sexual assault developed, considerable attention focused on establishing safeguards to protect men falsely accused of rape rather than protecting the victims of sex crimes. Only within the past 35 years have women been able to change those laws.

Despite progress in changing laws, traditional attitudes toward rape remain. Many people still believe that a victim must struggle physically for an attack to be classified as rape, that many victims are to blame for their own rapes, and that women who have had sex or have had sex frequently cannot bring a charge of rape. False beliefs like these are classified as rape myths.

VICTIMS LEGALLY UNABLE TO CONSENT

A victim is considered legally incapable of consenting to sexual activity if he or she, at the time of the rape, is mentally incompetent, **intoxicated**, drugged, or below the **age of consent**. Depending on the state, the age of consent varies from 14 to 18 years of age. If someone who is below the age of consent has sex with a partner who is older, the partner can be charged with **statutory rape**. Sex with someone who is under the age of consent is considered rape under all circumstances, and the minor's consent is not relevant in court.

Q & A

Question: I am below the age of consent in my state, but my mother knows I'm having sex with my boyfriend, and she says it is okay. Is it still against the law?

Answer: Your mother's consent does not make any difference. Your parents do not make the law. Just as there are laws governing teens in smoking, drinking, and driving, there are laws about the legal age of consent for sex. The age of consent laws always applies, regardless of whether you are in love, have been together for a long time, or have had sex before. Age of consent laws also apply to gay men and lesbians.

LEGAL REFORMS

Issues surrounding legal definitions of rape have been fiercely debated in the United States. In recent years, feminist groups have had some success in expanding the rights of victims.

Resisting rape

Many states once required that victims prove they had physically resisted an attack by showing signs of injury. Most state laws no longer require such evidence.

Rape shield laws

In the 1970s, under pressure from activists, lawyers, and legislators, most states enacted rape shield laws to ease the emotional burden of rape victims who testified in court. These laws limit the use of a victim's prior sexual history, which defense lawyers have used in the past to undermine a victim's credibility. Today, every state, including the District of Columbia, has a rape shield law. In 1978, the U.S. Congress added a similar provision to the Federal Rules of Evidence. Rule 412 declares that evidence offered to prove that a victim engaged in other sexual behavior or to prove a victim's sexual predisposition is generally not admissible in any civil or criminal proceeding involving alleged sexual misconduct.

As a result of these laws, the prosecution cannot usually introduce evidence of the victim's prior sexual history or reputation in court. It is no longer assumed that a woman consented to sexual intercourse because she has had sex in the past. However, because laws differ from state to state, some states still allow more testimony about the victim's past than others.

Most people recognize that allowing questioning about a victim's prior sexual history works against the victim and that the fear of being humiliated in court discourages victims from reporting the crime and pursuing charges. When such questioning is allowed during a trial, the jury's attention may be wrongly diverted away from the issue of the assailant's guilt by instead putting the victim on trial for her sexual past. Many people assume that without the protections afforded by rape shield laws, fewer cases would be reported, fewer cases would be prosecuted, and rapes and other sexual assaults might go unpunished. According to the National Center for Victims of Crime, rape shield laws were designed, in part, to make it more likely for victims to come forward. If rape victims are likely to have their entire sexual history revealed and examined in court as part of a rape prosecution, they may be deterred from reporting the crime against them. Although rape shield laws protect the victim against the introduction of such evidence during a trial, the laws do not protect victims from pretrial publicity.

On the other hand, there are people who think the rape shield laws are no longer necessary. It is especially common to hear arguments against rape shield laws in highly publicized date rape cases. Many argue that because premarital sex and other sexual activity are considered less shameful today, shield laws serve no function. Some people believe that the rape shield laws keep an accused rapist from receiving a fair trial and that the law discriminates against men. Such views are especially common in cases where a victim has a history of false accusations.

Recently, a 2007 study by researchers at the University of California, San Diego, examined the basic premise of rape shield laws. Namely, they examined whether or not women with extensive sexual histories were more or less likely to accuse a man of rape. If women who were very sexually active were more likely to make an accusation of rape, whether or not a rape had occurred, then it is possible that rape shield laws would actually be doing the accused a disservice. The scientists, however, found the opposite to be the case when they showed various types of women different scenarios of forced and **consensual** sex. Women who had extensive sexual histories were actually less likely to accuse their hypothetical partners of rape both when, in the scenario, an actual rape had occurred and when, in the scenario, no rape had occurred but they were given a strong motive for revenge. Moreover, women were much less likely to accuse a man of rape if, in a scenario, they had consented to extensive sexual contact with him in the past. This study gives strong support to the use of rape shield laws because the type of sexual history most likely to prejudice a jury against a victim actually seems to make women less likely to accuse their attackers, either falsely or justly.

Fact Or Fiction?

If a woman goes to a man's dorm room or house, she risks a sexual assault. If something

happens later, she can't claim that she was
raped because she should have known not to go
to those places.

The Facts: The "assumption of risk" wrongfully places the responsibility of the offender's actions on the victim. Even if a woman goes voluntarily to a man's home or room and engages in some sexual activity, it does not mean that she has consented to all sexual activity. She has the legal right to say "no" or "stop" at any point in the encounter.

Intimate partner rape

It is a crime if your boyfriend or other intimate partner has sex with you against your will. This is true even if you willingly had sex with him in the past. It is also a crime for a date or acquaintance to force you to have sex or coerce you into sexual activity against your will.

Similarly, another important legal reform has been the enactment of laws making marital rape a crime. Fewer than 30 years ago, a man could not be charged with raping his wife. Today, in all 50 states, courts recognize that an individual has the right to refuse to have sex even within the context of marriage.

See also: Date Rape; Statutory Rape

■ MALE ROLE IN RAPE

The World Health Organization (WHO) noted in its 2002 World Report on Violence and Health that "most acts of sexual violence are experienced predominantly by women and girls and perpetrated by men and boys." Data from the U.S. Department of Justice in 2005 found that 92 percent of rape and sexual assault victims over the age of 12 were female and 97 percent of rapes with single offenders were committed by males. Furthermore, more than 90 percent of multiple offender sex crimes also included at least one male attacker.

WHY SOME MEN RAPE

What drives one person to sexually assault another? Some anthropologists seek answers by examining other societies. In a 1981 study

DID YOU KNOW?

Risk Factors for Sexual Violence

Individual level

- Men using alcohol or drugs
- Men holding attitudes and beliefs supportive of sexual violence, including coercive sexual fantasies and blaming women for arousing them
- A pattern of behavior that is impulsive, antisocial, and hostile toward women
- Having been sexually abused as a child

Family and close environment level

- Growing up in a family environment characterized by physical violence, little emotional support, and few economic resources
- Associating with sexually aggressive peers

Community level

- Poverty, masculine identity is in crisis
- Weak sanctions against men who are sexually violent

Societal level

- Community and social expectations that women are responsible for protecting their modesty and controlling their sexuality
- Community and societal norms of male superiority and male sexual entitlement
- High levels of all forms of violence in a society
- Societies where laws and policies related to gender equality and sexual violence are weak

Source: World Report on Violence and Health, World Health Organization, 2002.

published in the *Journal of Social Issues,* a study that significantly influenced later research, anthropologist Peggy Sanday examined 156 tribal societies, classifying them as "rape-prone" or "rape-free." Rape-prone cultures separated the genders, gave less power to women, and had a higher rate of interpersonal violence than rape-free cultures. Many consider the United States to be a rape-prone society. The 1993 book *Rape: The Misunderstood Crime* revealed that at the time the United States has the highest rate of rape among industrialized nations. In a 2004 cross-national study of crime rate, researchers found that eight Western countries actually had the highest rape rate. However, it is very difficult to collect and compare sexual violence data from multiple nations.

Other researchers suggest medical reasons are behind sexual aggression. A 1988 study by Canadian psychiatrists published in the *Annals of Sex Research* reported that as many as 40 percent of sexually aggressive men had impairments in the right temporal lobe of the brain. There may also be a genetic predisposition to sexual coercion. In a 2008 study in Finland published in *Aggressive Behavior,* researchers found that part of the association between sexual coercion and alcohol use may be the result of a common genetic factor.

Returning to 1988, a group of psychologists published a study in the *Annals of the New York Academy of Science*. Trying to find ways to predict sexual aggression, the group examined the attitudes and histories of 2,972 male students at 32 colleges and universities. Researchers found that men who were hostile and aggressive, showing no empathy or remorse, were more likely to commit sexually aggressive acts. The study also noted that teenage boys were responsible for 20 percent of rapes and 50 percent of cases of child sexual abuse.

A. Nicholas Groth, a therapist who worked for 15 years with more than 500 incarcerated sex offenders, is an authority on sexual aggression. In his book *Men Who Rape: The Psychology of the Offender*, he describes three kinds of rapists: the power rapist, the anger rapist, and the sadistic rapist. Power rapists like to control their victims. Anger rapists are angry with women and can become brutal in their attacks. Sadistic rapists get a thrill out of mistreating their victims. Federal, state, and local law enforcement agencies use an expanded version of these descriptions in their efforts to prevent rape and capture perpetrators.

SOCIALIZATION

Socialization is the process of learning the many things individuals must know in order to become acceptable members of a society. Among the things individuals learn is what it means to be male or female in a society. Many Americans have strong feelings about the roles of men and women in society. When a young male is aggressive or destructive, people will often say, "boys will be boys." If a young female shows similar aggressiveness, people may scold her for being "unladylike."

Fact Or Fiction?

Rape happens because some men have powerful sex drives.

The Facts: Rapes are acts of violence, not acts of passion. The National Violence Against Women Survey jointly run by the National Institute of Justice and the Centers for Disease Control and Prevention found that 22 percent of female victims and 48 percent of male victims identified in the study had suffered their first rape before the age of 12. The fact that an adult or adolescent attacker would have a much easier time subduing a child suggests that physical strength drives a number of attacks.

A 2002 article in the journal *Sex Roles* examines several decades of research on the subject. While young males are taught to be manly, which may include being adventuresome, participating in team sports, and being aggressive (even in romantic or sexual matters), girls are encouraged to be "feminine"—quiet, agreeable, and passive. Similarly, "ladies" are not supposed to be interested in sex. These separate expectations are often referred to as a "double standard," one code of behavior for men and another for women.

As they grow up, young boys (and girls) are bombarded with societal messages about the way they are expected to act by parents, teachers, and the media. Often, the messages are unspoken. They can be found in the way one's father and mother interact. They can be found in family plans—creating a college fund for a son while expecting a daughter to marry rather than pursue higher education.

Q & A

Question: How does rape affect the people involved?

Answer: Both the victim and the perpetrator face negative effects from an act of rape. The victim must heal both physically and psychologically. If female, the victim also will worry about becoming pregnant.

The perpetrator will have to face accusations that can lead to being convicted of this serious crime and serving prison time. Both will face legal fees and may receive unwelcome media attention. Friends and relatives may shun both the victim and the perpetrator. Their lives may never be the same.

Cultural messages and expectations affect different people in different ways. The general message might be that boys are "entitled" to more because they are boys. However, because of social status, physical strength, or athletic prowess, some may take that basic message of entitlement and go farther.

A 1998 study in the *Psychology of Women Quarterly* examined the way attitudes about the roles played by the two genders work together. The researchers found that men held a wide variety of beliefs about masculinity. Traditional beliefs—ideas like male dominance and entitlement—play a part in forming attitudes as do a person's social status and acceptance or rejection of violence. Men who have traditional ideas about gender roles and who believe violence is an acceptable way of settling differences of opinion could be expected to engage in acts of sexual aggression.

TEENS SPEAK

I Knew She Wanted It

When I was a high school senior, I started dating a girl I really liked named Sharon. Sharon had been giving out lots of hints that she wanted to have sex with me. From the way she talked sometimes, I figured she'd have sex with anybody. She did have a fine body.

I waited for just the right time. Her parents were away, and I gave her a ride home. She invited me into the house, talking about homework, but I knew what it was really all about. I talked a little, then I made my move.

When I kissed her, Sharon started to act like she was afraid or something—I thought she was trying to make herself look good, behaving like a good girl.

> She cried and asked me to stop but there was no way I
> could. When she told me that it was her first time, I realized
> why she was so scared. By then, though, I couldn't stop.
> We never spoke again.

SITUATIONAL FACTORS

Circumstances sometimes affect the choices people make, resulting in their doing things they normally would never do. Consider the effects of alcohol. The National Violence Against Women Survey, a 1992 study by the National Institute on Drug Abuse, found that 75 percent of male college students and 55 percent of female college students involved in date rape had been drinking or using drugs. A more recent 2005 study found that very little had improved over time. Almost half of all rapes that took place on campus were attacks on women who were incapacitated by alcohol or drugs that they had chosen to consume.

In 2000, the National Institute of Justice released a report, *The Sexual Victimization of College Women*. Researchers found that of the 4,446 women surveyed, 1.7 percent had experienced a completed rape, and 1.1 percent had experienced an attempted rape in the six months since the beginning of the school year. Compare those percentages to figures obtained in a 1992 study of college sorority women reported in the journal *Sex Roles*. Among these females, 17 percent had been raped and 24 percent had experienced an attempted rape. Almost half of these attacks took place in a fraternity house. It is difficult to determine whether or not the rate is actually going down, or if lower assault rates in the National Institute of Justice report just reflected the particular phrasing of the question—attacks in the first six months of the school year. A 2005 study of students at two large regional universities found that 19 percent of women on campus had experienced a completed or attempted rape. Fraternity members accounted for a disproportionately large number of their attackers as well, namely 28 percent of the rapists in attacks where the woman was incapacitated by drugs or alcohol and 14 percent of the rapists where force was involved.

College fraternities have been notorious for tolerating and even encouraging dating violence. Studies have covered this situation for more than 20 years. A 1996 study published in the journal *Gender and Society* discusses a fraternity's "rape culture." The study was held on a campus where fraternities and sororities dominated the social scene. Researchers compared four fraternity houses identified as high-risk areas for women to four fraternities that students considered "safe."

The high-risk fraternities fostered an attitude that was hostile to women. They actively discouraged members from developing monogamous relationships. "Hooking up," brief (often one-night) connections were preferred, with the aim of having sex and moving on. Parties at high-risk fraternities were rowdier, with heavy drinking and overt sexual displays. Parties at the safer fraternities had more public displays of affection. Safer fraternities were also more likely than high-risk houses to have participated in rape prevention programs.

A 2000 study by the Harvard School of Public Health examined college alcohol use, discussing the phenomenon of binge drinking. The study defined binge drinkers as male students who had five or more drinks and female students who had four or more drinks in a row at least once in a two-week period. Researchers found that one of the strongest predictors for binge drinking was membership in a fraternity or sorority. Four of five students living in fraternities and sororities were binge drinkers. Similar results were found in a 2006 study of more than 3,000 members of one national fraternity and found that 86 percent of them were binge drinkers.

The Harvard study also reported that one of the effects of binge drinking was an increased risk of rape. Among binge-drinking females, 10 percent reported being raped or experiencing nonconsensual sex. Among non-bingeing females, only 3 percent reported a similar assault. These results have been confirmed by several further studies. One published in 2006 by the *Journal of School Health*, in which researchers looked at high school students in Hawaii, found that 15 percent of binge-drinking teens had experienced dating violence, compared to 5 percent of nondrinkers and 8 percent of other drinkers. Another study, which looked at adolescent girls across the country, also found that binge drinking was associated with a threefold increase in risk for a sexual attack.

The Harvard study found that athletes binged more than others. Among athletes, 29 percent engaged in binge drinking, compared to 20 percent in the general student population. College sports teams are another rape-prone social group. In recent years, many sports programs, including the University of Colorado football team, have faced accusations of sexual assault.

The problem is not new. A 1995 article in the *Journal of Sport and Social Issues* reported that even though athletes comprised only 3.3 percent of the college population, they were responsible for 19 percent of sexual assaults on campuses.

Part of the problem may be that student athletes see themselves as privileged members of the community. They may also hold more traditional views, including a belief in many rape myths. A 2002 article in the *American Journal of Health Studies* examined the attitudes of 704 intercollegiate athletes from five different schools. The researchers found that several groups had a high acceptance of rape myths, including male freshmen and sophomore athletes and male athletes who played team sports like football or basketball as opposed to individual sports like tennis.

The "team player" mentality may offer some explanation as to why athletes may participate in gang rapes. A 1999 study of abusive behaviors by college athletes in the *College Student Journal* found that athletes were more likely to be involved in such situations than fraternity members or nonathletes. Additionally, players involved in contact sports may have more trouble restraining their aggression when under the influence of alcohol.

When athletes move on to professional sports, the resulting celebrity can further fuel sexual aggression. Sports stars such as Magic Johnson, Mike Tyson, and Wilt Chamberlain have bragged about their numerous sexual conquests. However, accusations of sexual assault or abuse have tarnished the images of athletes such as Tyson, as well as basketball star Kobe Bryant and Florida offensive lineman Carl Johnson.

The problem of sexual victimization does not end once women enter the military. Women in all branches of the service have been subject to sexual victimization ranging from harassment to rape. According to the 2007 Department of Defense Annual Report on Sexual Assault in the Military, there were 2,688 sexual assaults reported in 2007. However, it is assumed that the actual number of assaults was much higher. In addition to all of the reasons that civilians do not report sexual assault, in the military such reports have also been shown to be potentially damaging to a service person's career. This fact is reflected in the Restricted Reporting option open to service people, where they receive health care after an attack but the attack is not reported to either local law enforcement or the military command. A 2001 article in the *Journal of Consulting Clinical Psychology* examined three groups of naval recruits, 7,850 in all. Researchers surveyed the recruits to see if childhood physical or sexual abuse were predictors of rape activity. From the three groups, 11.3 percent, 11.6 percent, and 9.9 percent of the men reported committing rape prior to their military service. All of these men who were guilty of sexual or physical abuse also had problems with alcohol abuse and had been with a large number of sexual partners.

Many people still say, "It's a man's world." For too many people, being a man means emulating sports stars by being aggressive on the field and in sexual matters. Traditional attitudes are changing, however. As boys become men, they are learning that in American culture, sexual aggression and rape are not to be tolerated by society.

See also: Abusive Sexual Behavior; Date Rape; Drugs, Alcohol, and Rape; Gang Rape

FURTHER READING
Benedict, Jeff. *Out of Bounds: Inside the NBA's Culture of Rape, Violence, and Crime.* New York: HarperCollins, 2005.
Smith, Earl. *Race Sport and the American Dream.* Durham, N.C.: Carolina Academic Press, 2007.

■ PEDOPHILE
See: Children and Rape

■ PREVENTION OF RAPE: BEING PROACTIVE
Taking precautions and positive steps to ensure one's safety and decrease the likelihood of a rape is called being proactive. Anyone can be a victim of rape. Taking preventive measures by educating oneself about rape, learning rape prevention strategies, and identifying ways

to keep oneself safe both at home and away from home can reduce the risk of becoming a victim of rape.

Q & A

Question: Is it true that only attractive girls and women are raped? My older sister is overweight and says that she doesn't have to worry about being raped.

Answer: Rapists do not choose their victims for their sexual attractiveness. Rape is about power rather than passion. Statistics show that rape victims include girls and women of all ages, from the elderly to very young children.

EDUCATION

Learning about rape and rape prevention is a part of being proactive. Books like this one are key to the process of education. Most public libraries have a variety of resources on rape prevention (books, magazine articles, government publications, and pamphlets). Also, by searching on the Internet for the term *rape prevention*, anyone can access the Web sites of dozens of organizations that specialize in offering rape prevention advice. In addition, many community organizations—hospitals, community centers, and mental health groups—offer special programs about rape and rape prevention.

Many neighborhoods or towns also have rape crisis centers that offer services to victims of rape. Although everyone hopes to never need those services, part of being proactive is being aware, without a crisis, of all of the resources that are available in one's community. Rape crisis workers typically provide support, legal advice, and counseling to rape survivors. To find out what resources are available in any community before they are needed, call a local hospital. Being proactive means being prepared.

LOWERING YOUR RISK

Education is only one step in being proactive. Other steps involve making changes in one's behavior and lifestyle, both at home and away from home.

DID YOU KNOW?

Rape Rates in the United States

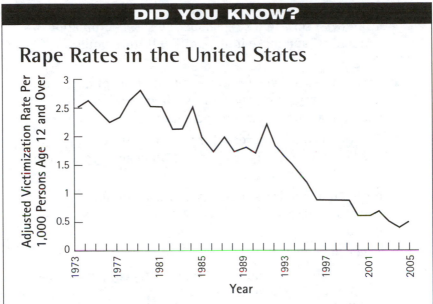

The decline in rape rates after 1993 coincides with the increased effort nationwide to educate the public about rape and rape prevention.

Source: National Crime Victimization Survey, U.S. Department of Justice, Bureau of Justice Statistics, 2006.

On the street

Many people begin by becoming more aware of their surroundings. They pay attention to what is happening around them. They use the following tips to increase their safety:

- When walking in an area where there are few people, avoid listening to the radio or other music because it will make you less able to hear what is happening around you.

- Make it a habit to walk with confidence and a sense of purpose. Police officers emphasize that rapists often prey on people who appear timid, uncertain, and aimless.

- Walk in well-lit areas when you have to be out at night.

- Never walk alone at night.

■ Avoid alcohol and drugs. These substances decrease awareness, slow reflexes, hamper muscle coordination and agility, and make it more difficult to respond to danger.

■ Do not use shortcuts or detours at any time of day that take you through empty areas, such as parking lots, alleys, abandoned lots, or wooded areas.

■ Do not walk, jog, or ride a bike alone in secluded areas. If you exercise regularly, on occasion change your route or time of your workout.

■ If someone in a car stops to talk or ask you for directions, keep your distance. Do not move closer to the car.

■ Never hitchhike.

■ If a car approaches and you feel threatened, scream and run in the opposite direction.

■ If someone approaches you on the street and no other people are around, do not stop and talk to that person. Keep walking. If he or she follows you and you feel threatened, scream or yell loudly, and move as quickly as possible to the nearest area where there are people.

■ When friends drop you off at home, ask them to wait until you are safely inside.

■ Have a key ready as you approach your home so that you can enter quickly.

At home

Many people believe that they are safe inside their homes. Yet the truth is that rape often occurs at home, largely because most people are raped by someone they know. Despite this fact, **stranger rape** also occurs at home. The following tips can reduce the risk of rape at home:

■ Avoid being at home alone with people you do not know or trust. If you must be at home with someone who fits this description, ask one or more friends to come over.

- Do not automatically open the door after you hear a knock. Ask people to identify themselves. If you do not know the person and you are home alone, do not open the door.

- Either on the phone or at the door, never reveal that you are home alone to people you do not know well.

- Do not allow a service person to enter your home unless you are expecting him or her.

- Talk with your parents about improvements that can make your home safer. Police experts recommend that a one-inch deadbolt lock be added to all entryways. They also suggest that all entryways and walkways be well-lit and all external doors and windows be locked. Security experts make these recommendations, not only to protect people from rape, but also to prevent other types of assault and burglary.

In the car

- Before opening the car door, check the interior of your car, including the front and back seats.

- Lock car doors immediately upon entering the car.

- Never pick up hitchhikers or other strangers.

- If possible, carry a cell phone whenever you drive or ride in a car.

- If you know you will be returning to your car when it is dark, park in an area that will be well-lit when you return.

- As you approach your car, scan the area from a distance. If one or more individuals are loitering near your car and you feel unsafe, return to a safe area. Wait for them to move. If they remain near your car, call the police.

- If your car breaks down and you are unable to phone for help, raise the hood and then get back in your car and lock the doors. If someone offers to help, do not roll down your window or open the door. Ask the person to call the police or roadside assistance for you.

Fact Or Fiction?

If you follow the rape prevention guidelines carefully, you can definitely protect yourself from being raped.

The Facts: As important as rape prevention strategies are to maintaining your safety, they cannot completely eliminate the possibility that you will be attacked or raped. On the other hand, law enforcement experts, security analysts, and rape counselors emphasize that rape prevention strategies are effective in decreasing the likelihood of rape.

SELF-DEFENSE

In a sense, every prevention tip is a form of self-defense—strategies that help people defend themselves against a sexual assault. Yet, in the field of crime prevention, the term self-defense also applies to specific programs that train one to fight back when physically attacked.

All of the martial arts—karate, judo, jujitsu, and others—teach people how to defend themselves against all kinds of crime, including rape. One disadvantage is that time and practice are necessary to become proficient and able to successfully defend oneself. As a result, several practitioners of the martial arts have developed self-defense training programs that require less instruction time, money, and practice but are as effective at providing self-protection as the martial arts.

A self-defense training system that many colleges and universities provide to their students is Rape Aggression Defense (RAD). Larry Nadeau, a karate master, former Marine, and police officer, designed RAD to teach women the importance of awareness, rape prevention techniques, and physical self-defense, including easy-to-learn martial arts tactics. In approximately nine hours, students learn enough to make them as proactive and as safe from rape as the experts maintain it is possible to be.

Another popular program is called Model Mugging. Martial arts expert Matt Thomas, who has studied 27 different forms of the martial arts, created the program in 1972 after a female karate expert was raped and beaten by an assailant. Thomas developed Model Mugging to help women physically defend themselves from attackers. Thomas tried to determine why karate was ineffective in the karate master's rape case. After studying rape victims and how they are attacked and rendered helpless, he decided that victims need strategies that will help them fight off an attacker who is lying on top of them. He then designed physical self-defense tactics to deal with this situation.

Like RAD, Model Mugging requires less time and money than is necessary to learn a martial art. A Model Mugging course typically runs about 20 hours.

TEENS SPEAK

I'm the Daughter of a Rape Victim

My mother was raped when she was 16; that's the age I am now. My aunts used to worry that her experience would make my mother overprotective. They were afraid that she might not let me go out at night or go out on dates. But that hasn't been my mother's reaction. She wants me to be independent and enjoy a social life. What has made a difference, I think, is that she is very involved in rape prevention.

My mother is a volunteer at the local rape crisis center. She had special training so that she can counsel rape victims and help them in the days and weeks after they've been raped.

From the time I was old enough to do things on my own, she has taught me to be careful around strangers and when I'm away from home. She also taught me that most women are raped by people they know. She has brought home pamphlets from the rape crisis center that give tips on how to avoid date rape as well as stranger rape. We read and discuss this information, and she encourages me to ask questions. Now we're both teaching my younger sister how to be smart and protect herself.

EDUCATING FRIENDS

Part of being proactive is making one's environment a better and safer place to live. Friends are an important part of that environment, and their words and behavior affect the quality of one's own life.

Remind your friends of the rape prevention strategies you learned and explain why you use those strategies when you are together. For example, when you suggest avoiding a shortcut through the woods at night and taking a longer but well-lit route, you are educating your friends and helping them become proactive.

If you see a friend drinking or taking drugs at a party, remind them that their safety depends on their ability to think clearly. Similarly, if you sense that a friend is headed for trouble with a date or an acquaintance, tell your friend that you are uneasy and are concerned for his or her safety.

Encourage your friends to learn more about rape prevention with you. Go to the library together or attend a community rape prevention program together.

PARTICIPATING IN COMMUNITY EFFORTS

Another important part of being proactive is improving the overall safety of one's community. Helping friends to become proactive is part of that goal. Another part is helping people in the community take rape prevention seriously.

Contact your local hospital, social service agencies, mental health clinic, and police to find out what rape prevention resources are currently available in your community. If you discover that there are very few or no services, ask your guidance counselor if he or she would be willing to invite rape prevention experts to talk to students. You might also ask the administrators of a local hospital or the leaders of civic organizations in your community to set up a prevention program. Follow up to see that they do.

See also: Date Rape; Drugs, Alcohol, and Rape; Educating the Community; Prevention of Rape: Being Reactive; Rape Within Abusive Relationships; Safe Areas, Establishing; Sexual Assault, Types of

FURTHER READING

Friedman, Jaclyn, and Jessica Valenti. *Yes Means Yes: Visions of Female Sexual Power and A World Without Rape.* New York: Seal Press, 2008.

Lindquist, Scott. *The Essential Guide to Date Rape Prevention.* Naperville, Ill.: Sourcebooks, 2007.

Slaughter, Lynn. *Teen Rape.* Detroit: Gale Group, 2004.

■ PREVENTION OF RAPE: BEING REACTIVE

Taking precautions to ensure one's safety by using one or more strategies to stop a sexual assault from progressing to rape. Being prepared to ward off a potential assailant is essential in preventing rape.

STRATEGIES TO STOP A RAPE
OR SEXUAL ASSAULT

Police officers, security analysts, rape counselors, and other professionals have identified actions a person can take to try to stop a rape. In doing so, they warn that every rapist and every act of rape is unique. A strategy that is successful in one case may not be in another situation. The key to using rape-stopping strategies is to remain calm and decide quickly which tactic is likely to be most effective and then use it firmly and decisively.

Q & A

Question: How do victims get the physical strength to fight back when attacked by a rapist?

Answer: When people are attacked, the brain responds quickly. Hormones, such as adrenaline, noradrenaline, and cortisol, are released into the bloodstream. The breathing rate and heart rate increase, causing blood to be pumped to the muscles, so that the body can physically respond to an attack. This physical reaction is called the "fight or flight response," and it gives people the strength to take action against a threatening situation.

If the rapist has no weapon

- Say "no" in a strong voice. Say, "This is rape." Sometimes if a rapist is told what he is doing, he will stop, particularly if the rapist is a date, a boyfriend, or someone you know. This strategy is also effective when used on an offender who is intoxicated.

- Find a way to escape. The best defense is to leave the scene as quickly as possible and to run as fast as you can to an area where there are other people.

- Scream and yell as loudly as you can. Yelling "fire" and "police" is more effective in attracting attention than yelling "rape."

- If the rapist is holding you and preventing your escape, attack him physically. If you take this route, make sure that the blows you deliver are forceful and strong. (A weak attack may only make the rapist angrier.) The pain from your attack must incapacitate the rapist for several moments or longer, giving you the time to escape.

- If you cannot get away from the rapist, vomit, urinate, or defecate, if possible. These behaviors sometimes cause rapists to leave the scene.

TEENS SPEAK

I Can Scream

In health class, we talked about all of the ways that a person can stop a rape when someone attacks. The teacher talked about kicking, hitting, and many other physical things you can do to escape from a rapist.

The problem is, I don't see how kicking or hitting is going to protect me from most people. That's because I'm not even five feet tall, and I only weigh 92 pounds.

After class, I told my friend what I was worried about. She reminded me that I have something that no one else has. She called it "my ear-piercing shriek that makes the blood run cold." I smiled because I knew it was true. I not only have a high-pitched scream, but I also have a really loud voice.

I felt a lot better realizing I had something that might help me if I'm attacked. It made me realize that everyone needs to think about their strengths and abilities in deciding which strategies will most likely work for them.

If the rapist is armed

If the rapist has a weapon, your options are limited. If you physically attack the rapist, he might use the weapon and rape you.

- Scream or yell "fire" or "police," unless the rapist threatens you with the weapon.

- If you know martial arts or have had self-defense training and feel confident that you can disable your attacker, you may wish to go ahead, but realize that you are taking a risk.

- If your attacker allows you to speak, tell him one of the following lies: You are menstruating and therefore are bleeding heavily or you are infected with HIV, herpes, or another STD. Or tell him that your father (brother, uncle, boyfriend) is coming soon. Sometimes these strategies deter rapists.

- When the rapist has a weapon, there is often nothing a victim can do to stop the assault. The most important action in these cases is to concentrate on surviving the attack and give in to the rapist's demands. Police experts recommend that you focus on memorizing the rapist's physical characteristics so that you can report him.

Fact Or Fiction?

Boys and men are stronger than girls and women and can fight off a rapist, even if the attacker has a weapon.

The Facts: Although boys and men have stronger muscles in their upper torsos and are often stronger physically than girls and women, this strength does not necessarily give them an advantage in an armed sexual assault. When a rapist is armed, every victim is equally at risk of being physically harmed by the rapist. Whether a victim is a girl or boy, man or woman, his or her response must take into consideration that the rapist may use the weapon, especially if provoked.

EVALUATING THE REACTIVE STRATEGIES

In selecting which strategy to use, quickly judge your attacker. Is the rapist drunk? If that is the case, then it is likely his thinking is unclear, his reflexes are slow, and he is not as coordinated as he usually is. Choosing a strategy that allows you to escape may be your best bet.

If a rapist is acting as if he thinks he is seducing you, vomiting or urinating will spoil his fantasy and make it less likely that he will continue. Telling him that you are menstruating or are pregnant may also stop him.

The "seducer" rapist may also believe you if you say you are strongly attracted to him and that you want to have sex with him. If you follow this conversation with the comment that you need to use the bathroom first, he may let you go.

Sometimes there is no "right" strategy or defense that will stop an attack, and nothing can be done to prevent the assault. If you are able to memorize the rapist's physical characteristics, you can later help the police locate and arrest him. By remembering as much as you can about the rapist, you can help make sure that he does not rape anyone else in the future. Among the characteristics you should memorize are:

- The rapist's car make and model, license number, and condition of the car
- Age, weight, and height
- Hair color and length
- Coloring (freckled, red-faced, tan, black)
- Eye color
- Clothing
- Facial hair
- Distinctive marks on his body, including scars, tattoos, body jewelry, body hair
- Type of body odor or other smell

IF YOU ARE A VICTIM OF RAPE

Rape victims often feel that they are to blame for an attack. Those who try reactive rape strategies and fail to escape often feel that they are at fault. They tend to believe that if they had tried harder, screamed louder, or kicked more, the rape would not have happened. Rape victims who were too paralyzed by fear to use a reactive strategy often feel guilty as well.

The truth is, no matter what happens, the victim is never to blame. The only person responsible is the rapist. Rape is an overwhelming, frightening **trauma**, a devastating emotional and physical injury. Sometimes nothing that a victim can do will be able to prevent or stop a rape.

The important thing to remember is that you survived a severe trauma. If you have been raped, you need to seek medical treatment. Ask a friend or family member to go with you to a hospital emergency room. The medical staff will treat your external and internal injuries, test you for sexually transmitted diseases (STDs), and help you decide what course you should take next.

See also: Date Rape; Help and Support; Prevention of Rape: Being Proactive; Sexual Assault, Types of

FURTHER READING

Denny, Todd. *Unexpected Allies: Men Who Stop Rape.* Victoria, B.C.: Trafford Publishing, 2007.

Feuereisen, Patti. *Invisible Girls: The Truth About Sexual Abuse—A Book for Teen Girls, Young Women, and Everyone Who Cares About Them.* New York: Seal Press, 2005.

Lindquist, Scott. *The Essential Guide to Date Rape Prevention.* Naperville, Ill.: Sourcebooks, 2007.

Warshaw, Robin. *I Never Called It Rape: The Ms. Report on Recognizing, Fighting, and Surviving Date and Acquaintance Rape.* New York: HarperPerennial, 1994.

Wiseman, Rosalind, and James Edwards. *Defending Ourselves: A Guide to Prevention, Self-Defense, and Recovery from Rape.* New York: Noonday Press, 1994.

■ RAPE

See: Law and Rape, The; Victims of Rape: Female; Victims of Rape: Male

■ RAPE AND RELIGION

Clergy members may offer support and counseling after someone is raped, but if they do not, victims should seek help and support elsewhere.

Q & A

Question: If a woman is raped, are there any drugs that could ensure that she not get pregnant?

Answer: Yes, emergency contraception exists, which is highly effective in preventing pregnancy if taken within 72 hours of unprotected sexual intercourse. Most hospitals will offer these drugs to rape victims. However, a Catholic hospital that follows the teachings against both contraception and abortion may not make exceptions to these prohibitions, even in the case of rape. Some Catholic hospitals offer emergency contraception and some do not. If someone is raped and wants emergency contraception, she should ask about it even if it is not offered at the hospital treating her. Most hospitals will direct a victim to where it is available, even if they will not provide it themselves.

THE CATHOLIC CHURCH, ABORTION, AND RAPE

The Roman Catholic Church holds that each **fetus** is a person from the time of **conception** and that abortion is therefore murder. There is no exception in this for a pregnancy that occurs as the result of rape.

Those who disagree with the official view of the Catholic Church, among others, argue that abortion is legal and safe. For many women, carrying a child that resulted from rape would be an excruciating reminder of the violence that was done to them. In addition, in cases of **incest**, there may be **genetic** or other health reasons not to carry a child to term. If someone is raped and a pregnancy results, the woman should speak to a rape crisis counselor, doctor, or religious adviser if possible, about all of the options available in order to make an informed decision about one's choices. Ideally, one of those options is emergency contraception. When taken within 72 hours of a sexual assault, emergency contraception is extremely effective in preventing pregnancy. For this reason, most Catholic hospitals do not encourage their doctors to provide emergency contraception to rape victims. Part of the reason is because the mode of action of emergency contraception is mixed; it can both prevent conception and stop a fertilized egg from implanting. The other reason is the general prohibition of contraception.

The U.S. bishops have formally issued a directive allowing doctors to provide emergency contraception to women who have been raped, as long as they test negative for an existing pregnancy. Unfortunately, despite the presence of this explicit permission from the Catholic Church, and the fact that emergency contraception can help a woman avoid choosing an abortion later on, there are still only a limited number of Catholic hospitals that offer emergency contraception to rape victims. Even fewer Catholic hospitals offer it to women in general.

SEXUAL ABUSE WITHIN THE CATHOLIC CHURCH

In the past few years, there has been a scandal in the Catholic Church regarding sexual abuse of children and others by Catholic priests. A study by researchers at John Jay College of Criminal Justice in 2002 found that about 4 percent of U.S. priests ministering from 1950 to 2002 were accused of sex abuse with a minor. The study reports that 4,392 clergymen, almost all priests, were accused of abusing 10,667 people, with 75 percent of the incidents taking place between 1960 and 1984. Court cases and settlements have cost the church hundreds of millions of dollars.

The John Jay study further found that an overwhelming majority of the victims, 81 percent, were males. The most vulnerable were boys ages 11–14, representing more than 40 percent of the victims. This goes against the trend in American society, where the main problem involves men abusing girls. Most of the accused committed a variety of acts involving serious sexual offenses. Those who were abused often kept silent for years and have suffered much anguish over harm inflicted by someone they trusted. In the years since the sexual abuse scandal among the Catholic clergy came into the public light, millions of dollars in restitution have been paid to abuse victims. In 2008, Pope Benedict XVI met with a small group of victims of clergy sexual abuse and offered them an apology for the horrible things they had experienced. During several large masses as well as in meetings with U.S. bishops, he also apologized for the problem of sexual abuse in the church and promised to do better.

JUDAISM AND RAPE

Ancient Jewish law both specifies fines for a man who rapes a woman and also demands that he marry her. However, in the modern world, Rabbinical courts are no longer qualified to enforce these laws. In modern cases of rape, a woman is generally presumed not to have consented to the intercourse, even if she consented after the sexual act began and declined a rescue. Judaism recognizes that forced sexual relations even within the context of marriage are rape and are therefore not permitted. Even Orthodox Judaism permits abortion if the mother's life is at stake.

ISLAM AND RAPE

Muslims tend to view women as subordinate to men, and views on rape can reflect this attitude. Women who report a rape are sometimes accused of sex outside of marriage, a serious crime in many Muslim societies. Aside from physical evidence that she resisted the rape and was injured in consequence, the only way to establish rape in some Muslim countries is by the testimony of four male witnesses (who must be Muslims in good standing) who actually saw the act itself. Without these witnesses and a confession from the accused rapist, the victim will be condemned by her very accusation: she wasn't raped; she participated in a sexual act outside of marriage. Women who are raped are sometimes seen as having brought shame to the family and are often discouraged by their families from reporting the crime.

Most Muslims believe that the soul enters the fetus when it is 120 days old. Therefore, abortion is often permitted under Islamic law until the fourth month, especially where the pregnancy is a result of rape or incest. After that time, however, most Muslims believe that abortion should only be permitted if the mother's life is in danger.

The decision about abortion following a pregnancy resulting from a rape is a complex and wrenching decision.

See also: Female Rights; Help and Support; Rape and Society; Rape in War

FURTHER READING

Bruni, Frank, and Elinor Burkett. *Gospel of Shame: Children, Sexual Abuse, and the Catholic Church.* New York: HarperPerennial, 2002.

■ RAPE AND SOCIETY

The structure of a society influences the frequency of sexual assault, including rape—or forced sexual intercourse—in that society. Numerous studies have been done that link various social characteristics to the likelihood that a woman will be raped. Several community factors have been shown to be strongly related to a country's prevalence of sexual assault.

The classic study of the effect of culture on rape was performed by the anthropologist Peggy Reeves Sanday in 1981. In her book *Female Power and Male Dominance: On the Origins of Sexual Inequality,* Sanday classified societies as either rape-free or rape-prone. Rape-free societies tended to be those in which women and men contributed equally to the community. They also tended to encourage children to value nurturing emotions and avoid aggression. In contrast, Sanday found that rape-prone societies had more separation of sex roles and that they tended to respect, or at least tolerate, male violence and aggression.

These results have been confirmed by other scientists. The 2005 World Health Organization (WHO) multicountry report on domestic violence and women's health found several societal factors that increased a woman's risk of **gender-based violence.** These include how equal men and women are economically, as well as confirming most of the other factors identified by Sanday in her groundbreaking work. One thing that the WHO report specifically mentions is that in societies where extended family and neighbors are unwilling to intervene in cases of domestic violence, domestic violence is more likely to occur. It is therefore important to speak out. Failing to act against violence is not just the tolerance of violence; it is the encouragement of violence.

In the words of the WHO report, "Challenging the social norms that condone and therefore perpetuate violence against women is a responsibility for us all." Rape, sexual assault, and all forms of violence against women may be crimes committed by individuals, but they are crimes shaped by society. Changing the way that societies view, and treat, women would be a more effective way of preventing gender-based violence than any amount of criminal prosecution.

VIOLENCE AGAINST WOMEN AND PUBLIC HEALTH

Since the early 1990s, the international community has recognized violence against women as a serious public health problem. A series of studies of 35 countries that was performed in the years leading up to 1999 found that between 10 and 50 percent of women had experienced violence at the hands of an intimate partner. Furthermore, between 10 and 30 percent of women and girls reported experiencing sexual violence at some point during their lives.

Violence is not only a tragedy in and of itself, but it also has a profound effect on a woman's health. In most countries, women who have ever experienced either physical or sexual intimate partner violence are significantly less healthy than their counterparts who have not been victims of partner violence. They experience not only reproductive health problems, such as increased risk of miscarriage, but also general health problems. Interestingly, any violence during a woman's lifetime is associated with recent reports of poor physical health. The effects of the violence remain long after the actual victimization has ended.

Intimate partner violence substantially increases a woman's amount of emotional distress. Women who have been the victims of partner violence are more likely to feel tired all the time, to cry easily, and to have difficulty enjoying life. They are also significantly more likely to experience thoughts of suicide.

TRADITIONAL GENDER ROLES

Men who strongly embrace traditional gender roles are more likely to commit rape. This has been shown in study after study. Men are more likely than women to believe that it is acceptable, or even expected, to pressure someone into sex or to blame the victim of an assault. However, men who exhibit the most traditionally masculine gender roles are even more likely to be sexually aggressive then men in general. Several scientists have found that men who are "macho" are more likely to say they would commit acts that would be considered to be rape or sexual assault.

One of the reasons that strong adherence to expected gender roles increases the likelihood of a man becoming a rapist is that the belief that people should behave in a certain way allows individuals to depersonalize their actions. If men are supposed to want sex and women are supposed to resist, then taking or demanding sex despite resistance is just what a man does if he is with a woman who says no. Following the expected behavior makes it less about the victimizer and the victim and more about something a "real" man is supposed to do.

Recently, researchers have tried to explain more of the nature of the association between adherence to traditional male gender roles and rape. Hill and Fischer, in a paper published in 2001, found evidence to suggest that the link might have to do with a sense of male entitlement. Many men, in particular men who adhere closely to masculine gender roles, feel they have a right to sexualize any woman they see. Furthermore, many also feel that they have a right to sex, particularly in situations where they believe they have provided a woman something of value. For example, a man may believe that a woman owes him sex if he has purchased her dinner or, even, simply if he has provided her with his company.

Men may also believe that they are entitled to sex if women lead them on by kissing or touching them. In other words, a man may believe that a woman is not entitled to change her mind about engaging in sexual intercourse or that any resistance after the woman has initially agreed to sexual contact is simply **token resistance.**

Finally, many men who strive to fulfill their masculine gender role expectations feel like being in a romantic relationship entitles them to sex. This may explain not only why in many date- and marital-rape situations, men do not necessarily believe they have done anything wrong, but also why these crimes often have lesser punishments and are seen as less serious than rapes by strangers or other forcible rapes.

MARITAL RAPE

It was only in 1993 that marital rape finally became illegal in all U.S. states. It was not until 2006, however, when the Violence Against Women Act of 2005 was signed into law that many states stopped officially treating marital rape as a lesser crime than rape with other types of victims. There are still, however, many individuals who believe that marriage is, among other things, a contractual obligation to provide sex and that, therefore, marital rape should not be treated in the same manner as even other intimate partner rapes.

Several countries were surveyed by the World Health Organization (WHO) multicountry study in which the vast majority of the women believed that there was never any circumstance in which it was acceptable for a woman to refuse her husband sex. In countries where a larger percentage of women thought that such refusals were at least sometimes acceptable, more women generally thought it was reasonable to refuse sex because they were sick than because they did not want sex or because their husbands were drunk or abusive. Although this view may seem extreme, it is not that different from the opinions of many individuals in the United States. Many studies have found that marital rape is seen by the general public as a less serious crime than other rapes. People even judge the severity of the rape based on the state of the marriage—seeing rape as significantly more serious even between individuals who are separated than between those who are still living in the same household.

UNDERSTANDING THE RAPE SCRIPT

There is a standard rape script, as portrayed in the media, which has very little relationship to how most rapes play out in real life. What people think of as rape is a violent, **nonconsensual** sexual assault by a stranger, frequently involving the use of weapons, where the victim is screaming her refusal. In reality, rapes rarely conform to that stereotype. Instead, most rapes are committed by individuals known to the victims, weapons are rarely used, and victims often end up giving in to their assailants out of fear or out of hope of avoiding confrontation.

A 2007 study by a group of German scientists looked at teenagers' understanding of typical events leading up to a first sexual encounter, both forced and consensual, and found some very interesting results. In a hypothetical situation where girls were assaulted in a manner dissimilar to the standard rape script but very similar to what often happens in real life, the girls were less likely than boys to consider it to be an assault. For example, such a hypothetical rape might include the aggressor getting his victim drunk so that she cannot object to having sex.

This is disturbing because it confirms numerous other studies that show that rape victims tend to be more susceptible to self-blame when rapes do not conform to the media pattern. When men coerce women into sex, through persistence, persuasion, alcohol or substance use, or other techniques but do not use violence, it is still an assault. It is extremely important that men and women learn that such techniques for acquiring sex are unacceptable and often against the law. Rape does not require violence. Rape is forcing someone to have sex without their consent, even if that force comes in the form of a type of verbal harassment, where the perpetrator simply continues asking for sex until the victim is too exhausted to keep saying no.

MEGAN'S LAWS

In 1994, a seven-year-old girl named Megan Kanka was raped and murdered by a known sex offender who lived down the street from her house. In the aftermath of the public outcry, federal legislation was passed to require that states not only register the addresses of sex offenders but also provide that information to the public. The state laws, which are collectively known as Megan's laws, allow individuals to determine whether sex offenders are living in their neighborhoods.

In 2006, Congress closed several loopholes in the sex-offender registration process by enacting the Adam Walsh Child Protection and Safety Act. This act requires all states to create publicly searchable Web sites that contain congressionally mandated, and standardized, information about local sex offenders. The goal of the act was to stop sex offenders from disappearing from the registry system by collecting standardized data and making the process more consistent and streamlined.

BLAMING THE VICTIM

Unfortunately, the trauma of a rape usually does not end when the attack is over. The victim is often not only forced to relive the attack, in her mind and during any law enforcement activities, but also to accept some blame for what happened to her. Despite the fact that the only person responsible for a rape is the attacker, often the victim receives some of the blame. This blame may be placed upon her by outsiders, including her friends and family, or by misplaced guilt present in her own mind.

One of the factors most associated with self-blame, as well as with the public's blaming the victim, is when someone is raped by a known assailant. Although this has become less of an issue over time, many individuals find it harder to believe that a woman has been raped if her attacker was her husband or another intimate partner. Even the woman herself is more likely to believe that she either did something to invite the attack or could have done something to prevent it.

Another factor associated with victim blaming and self-blame is willingness to engage in some level of sexual contact but not go all the way. Many individuals feel that men "can't stop" if they have gotten turned on to a certain degree and that, therefore, the woman is responsible for "leading them on" if she only wants to go so far. There is no factual or scientific basis for this belief. However, rape victims are more likely to experience blame if they say "no" after participating in some level of sexual activity, such as making out or heavy petting.

Finally, some individuals see anything that a woman does to make herself feel more sexually attractive, such as wearing a short skirt or a low-cut top, as equivalent to a sexual invitation. Therefore, they may believe that, given the presence of such an invitation, any sexual encounter with a woman who has gotten dressed up to attract men would not be rape. This is one way that individuals rank victims as more and less acceptable targets for attack. For individuals who have this kind of mind-set, it would be less of a crime to rape a woman who gets dressed up and goes to a bar than one who spends her evening studying in the library.

In the WHO multicountry study, scientists found that the extent to which women found violence acceptable varied from country to country. When presented with different scenarios and asked whether violence would be justified, depending on the country, between 6 and 80 percent of women thought violence against women was acceptable if a woman was unfaithful to her husband. Similar percentages of women thought violence was acceptable if women disobeyed their husbands, and up to approximately 65 percent of women thought violence was an acceptable response to a woman not completing her housework.

INTERNATIONAL WOMEN'S DAY

International Women's Day, a celebration on March 8 of the lives of women, was started by the United Nations (UN) in 1975. Two years later, in 1977, the UN General Assembly passed a resolution that stated that member countries should spend one day each year celebrating the United Nations Day for Women's Rights and International Peace.

Although International Women's Day is primarily about equalizing the role of women in society, doing so is, in and of itself, an important way to reduce violence against women. Women who live in societies that treat women as equal to men, that value their contributions, and that do not marginalize them to "woman's work" or otherwise limit their opportunities, are less likely to experience rape.

See also: Educating the Community; Female Rights; Rape in the Media, Reporting; Sexual Assault, Types of; Stigma of Rape

■ RAPE IN THE MEDIA, REPORTING

Accounts of sexual assaults in the media—newspapers, magazines, and on radio, television, and the Internet—tend to be highly selective, which can lead to misinformation. For example, news coverage often emphasizes rape by strangers even though most rapists are friends, relatives, or acquaintances. News reports may also sensationalize sexual attacks in ways that may be insensitive to the victim and the victim's family.

Q & A

Question: Is it against the law for a newspaper to publish the name of a rape victim?

Answer: It is not against the law. However, because of the nature of sexual crimes, most newspapers do not publish a rape victim's name out of respect for his or her privacy. Some people feel this custom creates a double standard since the name of the person accused of a sexual crime is published even though he or she has not yet been proved guilty in a court of law. These critics claim that a woman who has made false accusations in the past is free to do so time and again because as a potential victim, her identity will be protected. They also claim that the business of the media is to report as fully and accurately as possible and not make moral judgments about who should and should not be publicly identified. Finally, critics claim that by allowing rape victims to remain anonymous, the stigma of rape is perpetuated.

Although most media outlets do not release the names of rape victims, interviews with neighbors or relatives often provide enough revealing details that many people are able to recognize the victim. In addition, the media usually include only informational interviews with police and law enforcement. Although that perspective is relevant, other perspectives might provide more valuable information to the public. For example, experts on sexual violence (rape crisis center staff, counselors, prevention educators) could help dispel myths and correct misinformation. In addition, news coverage seldom alerts readers or viewers to local services available to victims of rape, sexual assault, and child sexual abuse.

Fact Or Fiction?

It doesn't matter what the media says about a rape case. After all, the accused assailant will still get his day in court.

The Facts: Unless a rape trial is moved far away from where it happened, media reports will affect the way potential jurors think about the case. For example, rape shield laws prohibit prosecutors from asking the victim too many questions about his or her past sexual activity. These laws are designed to not only protect the victim from unnecessary embarrassment but also keep jurors from deciding the case based on legally irrelevant information. If jurors have already learned from news reports information that is prohibited from court testimony, the trial may not be a fair one. On the other hand, testimony is usually not permitted about previous "bad acts" of the accused either. Again, if jurors already know these facts from news reports, the accused rapist may not get a fair trial.

INCREASED AWARENESS IN THE MEDIA

Although the media tends to sensationalize sexual assault cases, most outlets also reflect recent legal reforms. In covering some rape trials, for example, reporters help their audiences understand the idea that marital rape is possible or that victims are courageous for coming forward. The media has also highlighted a few highly sensational date rape cases, making us aware that date rape is a crime.

Most reporters do not have the background to understand the complexities of sexual assault cases. Like anyone, they also reflect the prejudices of society, and those prejudices affect how they report sexual crimes. In 2004, a study by researchers Park, Clark, and Gordon presented at the Association for Education in Journalism and Mass Communication considered whether sensitivity training would change the way that journalists covered domestic violence stories. The study found only a slight to moderate effect on coverage as a result of the training. For example, journalists who had the training were less likely to use statements that excused the assailant's behavior than those who did not.

ACCURACY OF REPORTING

Journalists hold biases that may affect how they refer to assailants or victims in their stories. The news media can also be selective in which cases they report and how they refer to those cases. For example, a study sponsored by the Department of Justice found that the ways in which the news media responded to studies depended on the results of those studies. When researchers found, for example, that domestic violence is predominantly perpetrated by men in order to exercise control over their female partners, some newspapers claimed that "feminist theorists" orchestrated a "myth-making industry" to promote "half-truths based on ideological dogma." On the other hand, when a few researchers found men and women to be equally guilty of committing battery, the researchers were labeled by some widely read newspapers as scientific "pioneers" pursuing hard facts and empirically sound data. In these cases, it is not that the reporting was necessarily inaccurate but that the information reported was characterized in ways that influenced public perception of a problem—sometimes in a misleading way.

To check news stories for inaccuracy or bias, figure out who the sources for the story are. Is the source someone you trust to give accurate information? From whose point of view is the story reported? Are other points of view represented? Do the media judge one group more harshly than other? For example, if the suspected assailant is a young man of color, is he referred to as a particularly dangerous predator? In what way is the report different from how a white man or an older man is referred to? Do stereotypes of certain groups skew news coverage of certain types of crimes?

IMPACT ON SOCIETY'S VIEWS

Over the past 40 years, a variety of legal reforms have afforded rape victims increased rights within the courtroom. As a result, more and more people have come to regard rapes and their victims as serious crimes. The media has played a major role in this change in public perception.

Prior to the early 1970s, the American legal system put the burden in rape cases on women. Any suggestion that a woman was sexually active outside of marriage was enough to nullify the charge of rape in the minds of many. By the 1970s, however, courts no longer put the victim on trial by introducing evidence of her past sexual history. Laws also began to rank sexual offenses. By doing so, prosecutors had a better chance of conviction in cases where the crime was legally shy of rape. For the first time, many states also passed marital rape laws.

During the 1970s, 1980s, and 1990s, several highly publicized cases introduced the public to new ways of thinking about sexual assault and rape. Although the news coverage was often less than ideal and only provided part of the story, the public did get at least a partial understanding of rape reform laws and the reasons underlying them. This coverage, in turn, increased understanding of rape and support for sexual assault victims. As more cases continue to be covered openly in the media, the public is more likely to recognize the complexity of behaviors that may constitute sexual assault.

See also: Educating the Community; Law and Rape, The; Rape and Society

FURTHER READING

Park, Ginger L., Terrie Clark, and Joye Gordon. *Effects of Domestic Violence Coverage Training on Student Reporting.* Chicago: Association for Education in Journalism and Mass Communication, 2004.

Taylor, Stuart, and KC Johnson. *Until Proven Innocent: Political Correctness and the Shameful Injustices of the Duke Lacrosse Rape Case.* New York: St. Martin's Griffin, 2008.

■ RAPE IN WAR

For thousands of years, wars have included sexual attacks, especially on women and children. In recent history, women have been sexually assaulted and tortured by opposing forces in areas as diverse as Bangladesh, Rwanda, and the former Yugoslavia.

Fact Or Fiction?

Rape in war is a new phenomenon.

The Facts: Rape has been used during war to terrorize and subjugate people throughout history. The Bible describes the rape of women who belonged to conquered tribes as a routine act. In medieval and early modern Europe, women of a besieged town were often raped. In World War II, Korean "comfort women" were forced into sexual servitude by the Japanese army. Thousands of Bengali women were sexually assaulted during Bangladesh's war of secession from Pakistan in 1971.

WHY ARE WOMEN RAPED IN WAR?

According to Amnesty International, women are raped because they are seen as "the reproductive machinery of the enemy" and the "embodiment of a community's honor." Rape becomes a military strategy—by attacking women, soldiers are attacking the morale of the enemy and humiliating not only the women themselves but also their men, who feel they have failed to uphold their honor. Rape is also used to terrorize the enemy, and sexual assaults in the context of war are often gang-related and sadistic.

EFFECTS OF RAPE IN WAR

Women who are raped during wartime may also experience the loss of home and community, injury, and untreated illnesses. Many have also witnessed the murder, injury, or rape of loved ones. The effects of these types of **trauma**, or emotional and physical shock, can be long-lasting and devastating. Many women who are raped suffer from **post-traumatic stress disorder (PTSD)**, a syndrome character- ized by the reexperiencing of the trauma in memories and dreams, avoiding anything reminiscent of the event, memory loss, emotional numbing, sleep disturbance, anxiety, severe depression, and alcohol and substance abuse.

The usual religious and cultural attitudes surrounding rape in a given culture can have further ramifications for women raped dur- ing war. For example, many Muslims believe the honor of a woman reflects upon her entire family. Therefore, some rape victims perceive their rape as punishment for some sin they may have unknowingly committed. Even if they do not blame themselves, they may feel so strongly about their responsibility to protect their family that they remain silent about the assault. Others speak out only to find that their families blame them for the rape or for bringing shame to the family, even if there was no way they could have avoided the attack.

For example, Amnesty International and other human rights groups have estimated that tens of thousands of people, mainly Muslim women and girls, were raped during the 1992–1995 war between the Serbs and the Bosnians in the former Yugoslavia. Many of the Bosnian rape victims remained silent or told very few people about what had happened to them due to the negative cultural and religious attitudes toward rape.

Other cultures also have social taboos around the issue of rape. In Sierra Leone, thousands of girls and women were raped—often for days or months on end and often by several men—during the civil war in that West African country in the 1990s. Because of social restrictions, these women and girls find it difficult or impossible to marry. Husbands and other family members rejected many of those who were already married. In contrast, some women from Nicaragua and other parts of Latin America expressed pride in having been raped in war because their political beliefs taught them that they have given their bodies to the revolution.

Systematic and widespread rape during war can also threaten the long-term health of women. Gynecological problems, including pain and infertility, can result. Sexually transmitted diseases can be passed on, including HIV and AIDS. In fact, in African conflict zones, according to a report released in 2004, rape as a weapon of war has created a humanitarian crisis for tens of thousands of women and girls and threatens to increase the spread of AIDS in the region. The report, *Rape, Sexual Violence and HIV in Conflict and Post-Conflict Zones*, by Women's Equity in Access to Care and Treatment, provides comparative case studies documenting sexual violence in Sudan, Uganda, Rwanda, Kenya, and the Democratic Republic of Congo. The report also calls for greater protection for rape victims from further sexual torture; access to emergency medical services, including postexposure **prophylactic, antiretroviral drugs**, which may help prevent AIDS from developing; rape counseling; and food and shelter.

The crisis in Darfur has once again brought the problem of rape during war to the public eye. Since 2003, more than 2 million individuals have been displaced from their homes, and rape has been used systematically as a weapon of warfare. Although the charge is considered to be somewhat controversial, in 2008 the International Criminal Court accused the president of Sudan of masterminding a program of rape as genocide against the people of Darfur. Many people believe that the Sudanese president is using rape as a method of ethnic cleansing, to rid the country of three ethnic groups that have challenged his power. One good thing has happened, however, as the result of the horrors of Darfur, the assaults committed by peacekeepers around the world, and the increase in violence against women seen in Zimbabwe. In 2008, the United Nations finally declared that rape and other forms of sexual violence constitute war crimes, and fighting these crimes received official priority.

Q & A

Question: Are there any laws against rape during war?

Answer: The Geneva Convention, ratified in 1949, which is the body of international law that governs behavior during times of war, states that "women shall be especially protected against any attack on their honour, in particular against rape, enforced prostitution, or any form of indecent assault." The Geneva Convention allows that a grave breech of its law can be punished in a country's national courts. It may also be possible to prosecute offenders in the international court found in The Hague, in the Netherlands.

See also: Law and Rape, The; Rape and Religion; Rape and Society

■ RAPE KITS AND EVIDENCE COLLECTION

A standardized kit containing the supplies necessary to collect evidence from a rape victim. Rape kits are designed to meet both medical and legal needs. They allow a trained provider to efficiently and effectively gather samples in a way that maintains the **chain of evidence** required to effectively **prosecute** a sex crime. A rape kit can only be assembled with the victim's **consent**. Even when a victim does not think she wants to prosecute her attacker, it is in her best interest to allow a rape kit to be completed in case she changes her mind later.

COLLECTING EVIDENCE USING A RAPE KIT

Sexual assault cases are unique, because in them the victim's body is itself a crime scene. Rape kits contain the instructions and supplies needed to collect evidence from the body that can assist in the prosecution of a sexual offender. Numerous types of physical evidence are collected as part of a rape kit. The mouth, vagina, and rectum are swabbed for bodily fluids that can be linked to the attacker. The victim's pubic hair and head hair are combed to collect any loose hairs that may belong to the attacker, and then samples of each are plucked for comparison. Fingernail clippings, and samples from underneath the nails, are collected in the eventuality that the victim scraped her assailant. Blood samples are also taken to test for drugs and alcohol, and the victim is thoroughly examined and photographed to document his or her injuries. Finally, each piece of the victim's clothing is bagged in individual paper bags so as to preserve any evidence, such as hair, skin cells, or fibers from the attacker's clothing, which may have stuck to it. All the collected evidence is then transported to the crime lab for eventual testing.

Q & A

Question: I need to know what I should do if I am ever sexually assaulted. How can I give the police the best chance of finding and catching my attacker?

Answer: First, it is important to go to a hospital emergency room (ER) as soon as possible after an attack. Some evidence can only be collected within the first 72 hours following the assault and, in general, sooner is better. If you think you have been given a rape drug, it is particularly important to get to the hospital as soon as possible because some such drugs are quickly **metabolized** out of your system and will stop showing up on tests.

Before you go to the hospital, do not shower, bathe, douche, brush your teeth, or clean your body in any other way. If you can avoid urinating or drinking before going to the hospital, that will help to preserve evidence as well. Ideally, you should go to the emergency room in the clothes you were wearing during the attack. If you cannot, place each piece of clothing into its own **paper**, not plastic, bag and bring the bags to the hospital with you. As soon as you can, you should also write down a description of what happened to you, including as much information as you can remember about your attacker.

Feel free to bring a friend with you to the hospital. You may also want to call your local rape crisis hotline. They can send a counselor with you to the hospital to make sure that you are treated properly and that evidence collection is done promptly and correctly.

A rape kit should be collected as soon as possible after the crime has taken place. This minimizes opportunities for loss of evidence, while allowing the victim to return to his or her life as quickly as possible. Since victims are instructed not to bathe, drink, urinate, or do any other activity that may disrupt the evidence on their bodies before the rape kit is performed, waiting for the procedure can itself be traumatic.

Although rape victims are usually sent to a hospital emergency room for treatment and evidence collection, ER doctors may not be the ideal people to collect a rape kit. They are often distracted by other patients who need urgent care. Studies have shown that some doctors also resent the several hours of time needed to properly complete a rape kit when it does not require their special skills. Furthermore, even doctors who sincerely want to help may be worried about collecting the kit incorrectly or having to spend time at trial. This is why many cities have rape crisis centers and specially trained personnel who can help speed the completion of a rape kit.

Victims and their family members should not try to collect evidence themselves or handle collected evidence. In order for the evidence to be useful in a court of law, specific procedures must be followed so that the police, lawyers, and judges know that the evidence has not been tampered with. For example, when evidence is collected, it is labeled not only with the victim's name and the type of evidence but with the collector's name. Then, everyone who handles the evidence must sign a piece of paper to document the chain of custody, even if they are only carrying it from one room to another.

Fact Or Fiction?

Only specially trained people can collect evidence for a rape kit.

The Facts: Not all doctors and nurses have been trained in how to collect a rape kit, and some may not even know that they should be doing one for any woman who comes in reporting a sexual assault. However, all hospitals should have access to rape kits, which contain instructions for properly collecting evidence. Following the instructions, and using the materials provided in the kit, allows even a relatively untrained individual to collect the evidence needed for a police investigation. On some college campuses, volunteers at rape crisis centers are trained in how to collect evidence for a rape kit so that they can accompany victims to the emergency room and make sure everything is done properly.

SANE

Sexual assault nurse examiners (SANE) are nurses who have been specially trained in dealing with sexual assault victims. Where SANE programs are available, these women are on call 24 hours a day, seven days a week, so that they can handle any sexual assault cases that are reported. By taking care of evidence collection and early treatment, including initial counseling, **emergency contraception** to prevent pregnancy, and sexually transmitted disease **prophylaxis,** SANE nurses free up valuable medical and police resources for care and investigation while giving sexual assault victims the most comprehensive care and protection available. SANE nurses are also generally more prompt about performing an exam than emergency room physicians, because they do not have to worry about other patients. In addition, they may have access to special equipment that allows them to perform more thorough rape kits—such as supplementing standard photography with **colposcopy** to document any vaginal or rectal tearing. Although there has been limited research in the area, studies suggest that rape kits collected by SANE nurses are more likely to be correct and complete compared to those collected by their less well-trained counterparts. Women treated by SANE nurses are also more likely to receive thorough counseling about pregnancy and STD risk than rape victims who are not treated by specially trained personnel.

THE UNPROCESSED RAPE KIT CONTROVERSY

Although rape kits are an efficient way to collect evidence, they are only useful if that evidence is eventually analyzed. Unfortunately, across the United States there is an enormous backlog of unprocessed rape kits. Due to a lack of resources in many cities, instead of rape kits being routinely analyzed, they are simply put away until

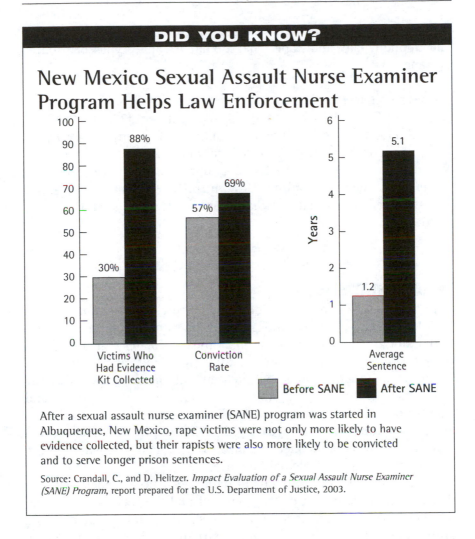

DID YOU KNOW?

New Mexico Sexual Assault Nurse Examiner Program Helps Law Enforcement

After a sexual assault nurse examiner (SANE) program was started in Albuquerque, New Mexico, rape victims were not only more likely to have evidence collected, but their rapists were also more likely to be convicted and to serve longer prison sentences.

Source: Crandall, C., and D. Helitzer. *Impact Evaluation of a Sexual Assault Nurse Examiner (SANE) Program*, report prepared for the U.S. Department of Justice, 2003.

and unless a specific suspect is located for comparison. To address the backlog, Congress proposed the Debbie Smith Act, named after a woman whose rape had been solved by DNA testing. The Justice for All Act, which passed in 2004, provided funding of $755 million to analyze unprocessed rape kits and related evidence. At the time the act was passed, Congress estimated that there were more than 300,000 unprocessed rape kits sitting on shelves around the country.

See also: Drugs, Alcohol, and Rape; Educating the Community; Help and Support; Law and Rape, The; Sexual Assault, Types of; Stigma of Rape

FURTHER READING
"Reference Card: Minors and Rape Crisis Treatment (2006)" New York Civil Liberties Union. Available online. URL: http://www.nyclu.org/rapecrisistreatment. Accessed December 2008.
"What Should I Do After a Rape?" Rape Abuse & Incest National Network. Available online. URL: http://www.rainn.org/get-infor mation/legal-information/what-should-i-do. Accessed December 2008.

■ RAPE STATISTICS

Rape statistics are the collection and interpretation of quantitative data (numbers) and probabilities (the chances of something happening). Using these numbers and probabilities, estimates can be made as to how whole populations may act. Statistics about rape are collected by numerous organizations and government agencies, including the Department of Justice (DOJ) and the Centers for Disease Control and Prevention (CDC). National surveys about crime and violence against women are conducted each year by the DOJ. Academic studies at colleges and universities sometimes also give valuable statistical information about rape and sexual violence.

Rape statistics are difficult to compile. The numbers change depending on the definition of rape used and the ways in which the numbers are gathered. Because rape is so often not reported to the authorities, crime statistics tell only part of the story. For example, the 2006 National Crime Victimization Survey found only around 41 percent of rapes had been reported to the police. This actually represents a significant improvement in reporting rates, but there is still a long way to go before crime statistics are anywhere close to showing the true scale of sexual violence that occurs in the United States. Also, rape and sexual violence differ greatly across different populations, so surveys do not tell the entire story. The statistics gathered in a survey are only accurate for that particular group being studied, and although some generalizations may be made, they may not tell us anything about other groups.

FACTS AND FIGURES

According to the National Violence Against Women Survey (NVAWS), one in six women and one in 33 men in the United States have experienced an attempted or completed rape at some time in their lives. Young women are at particular risk for sexual violence. A 1998 DOJ study found that 22 percent of rape victims were under the age of 12, 54 percent were under the age of 18, and 83 percent were under the age of 25.

Although by 2005, the DOJ was no longer publishing data for victims under the age of 12, the agency found that the rate of rape and sexual assault of individuals aged 16 to 19 was still almost three times higher than for those aged 12 to 15 or 20 to 24, and those rates were also substantially higher than that of any other age group. Older teenagers are at risk for the greatest rate of sexual assault of any age group.

This risk is supported by data from the Youth Risk Behavior Surveillance System (YRBSS), a national survey of high school students that is performed every two years. The 2005 cycle of the YRBSS found that, nationwide, 7.5 percent of high school students had been forced to have sexual intercourse. Rates were higher among girls, 10.8 percent, than among boys, 4.2 percent, and were also higher among black girls (11.5 percent) than white girls (10.8 percent), whose rates of experiencing forced intercourse were in turn higher than that seen in Hispanics (9.4 percent).

The Centers for Disease Control, which runs the biannual survey, also found that dating violence, in general, is also high among high school students. Almost 10 percent of students had been intentionally hit, slapped, or otherwise hurt by a boyfriend or girlfriend in the year preceding the survey. Such abuse was more common in black (11.9 percent) and Hispanic (9.9 percent) teens than in white teens (8.2 percent). Although the amount of dating violence in a given state varied from 6 percent to 16 percent, even the low end of the range represents a disturbing amount of violence among high school youth.

College students are at even higher risk. In 2005, the National College Women Sexual Victimization Study estimated that between 20 and 25 percent of college women experienced completed or attempted rape during their college years. Even younger children are not immune. A government study by the Department of Health and Human Services in 2003, based on a review of state records pertaining to child abuse and neglect, found that 86,830 children in the United

States experienced sexual abuse in 2001. By 2006, that number had decreased to 77,941.

Across all age groups, women are more likely to be victims of rape and sexual assault than men. Of the rapes and sexual assaults reported in the 2005 National Crime Victimization Survey, reported by the DOJ in 2006, 92 percent of the victims were women, and 8 percent were men. Women of color are also more likely to experience sexual assault. According to the NVAWS, in 2000, Native American and Native Alaskan women were more likely to report that they had been raped (34 percent) than any other group. Nineteen percent of African-American women reported they had been raped, as did 18 percent of white women. The 2005 National Crime Victimization Survey also found that African-American women were raped three times more often than white women and that multiracial women were even more frequently victimized.

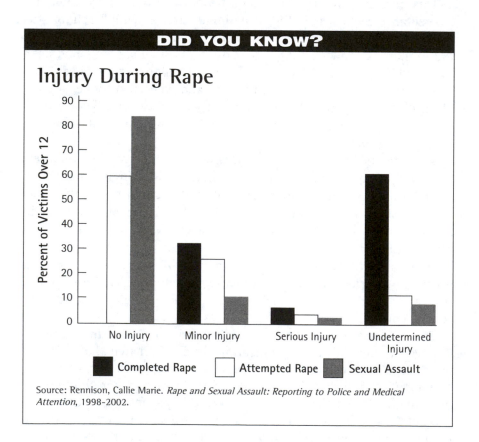

DID YOU KNOW?

Injury During Rape

Source: Rennison, Callie Marie. *Rape and Sexual Assault: Reporting to Police and Medical Attention*, 1998-2002.

Besides being of a young age, there are several other factors that seem to put someone at risk for sexual assault. In some cases, the relationship between these factors and sexual victimization is not always direct. For example, according to multiple studies, drug or alcohol use increases the likelihood of rape. This may be because alcohol and drug use lower inhibitions or because it makes someone less likely to be able to resist sexual aggression. However, it may also be true that drug and alcohol use may place women in settings where they are more likely to encounter potential perpetrators.

A prior history of sexual violence also puts victims at increased risk of future victimization. A study by researchers Tjaden and Thoennes that was conducted in the United States in 2000 found that women raped before the age of 18 were twice as likely to be raped as adults, compared to those without a history of sexual abuse. Many researchers believe that this may be a result of risk-taking behaviors brought on by psychological reactions to the original rape. Also, women with many sexual partners are at increased risk of experiencing sexual abuse. In short, having multiple partners is both something that makes one vulnerable to rape as well as something that is a consequence of prior sexual abuse.

Other statistics, according to Krug in 2002, for example, indicate that poor women are more likely to be the victims of sexual assault than are middle-class or rich women. Poverty may make the daily lives of women and children dangerous (for example, walking alone at night, less parental supervision) and put them at greater risk for experiencing sexual violence. In addition, poor women may be at risk for sexual violence because their economic status forces them into certain high-risk occupations, including prostitution. This is supported by data from the 2005 National Crime Victimization Survey, which found that the poorest women are at the greatest risk of rape and sexual assault.

Who are the perpetrators of sexual violence?

Most rapists are known to their victims. One study by Tjaden and Thoennes in 2000 showed that eight out of 10 victims knew the perpetrator, and, in most cases, the assailant was someone close to the victim. In the NVAWS, 64 percent of women and 16 percent of men reported being raped, physically assaulted, or stalked by an intimate partner, including a current or former spouse; a **cohabiting**, or live-in, partner, boyfriend, or girlfriend; or a date. Similarly, in the National Women's Study, intimate partners, which are current or former spouses or boyfriends, represented 19 percent of perpetrators; family members represented 27 percent of perpetrators; and 29 percent were relatives, friends, or acquaintances. Only 22 percent of perpetrators were strangers. The percentage of stranger assaults was slightly higher according to 2005 Department of Justice statistics—31 percent—but it is possible that intimate partner assaults are less frequently reported to the police.

Fact Or Fiction?

You can avoid being raped if you do not go out at night.

The Facts: Most women who are raped are raped by someone they know, *not* by a stranger. According to the Department of Justice, 67 percent of women raped or sexually assaulted in 2005 by a single offender were victimized by a spouse, ex-spouse, partner, friend, acquaintance, or relative. Only a small percentage of rapes are perpetrated by a stranger. Therefore, you cannot protect yourself completely from sexual assault simply by avoiding strangers while out at night.

Also according to Krug and other researchers in 2002, individuals with the following characteristics are more likely to commit rape or other acts of sexual violence:

- Alcohol and drug use
- Coercive sexual fantasies (fantasies of forcing sex on someone)
- Impulsive and antisocial tendencies (can't or won't control their impulses)
- Preference for impersonal sex
- Hostility toward women
- History of sexual abuse as a child
- Witnessed family violence as a child
- Associates with sexually aggressive and delinquent peers
- An emotionally unsupportive family environment

Many sex offenders begin a pattern of violence at an early age. In one study in 1993, Shaw and others found that the majority of sexual offenders reported assaulting someone before they were 18 years of age. Approximately 20 percent of all rapes and 30–50 percent of child molestations are by youths under the age of 18. The average juvenile offender has committed eight–nine sexual offenses and averaged four–seven victims. These young people often continue to commit crimes as they age. In a 2006 study from the *Journal of Interpersonal Violence,* researchers examined repeat offenses by sex offenders who had committed their first assault while they were still teenagers. They found that juveniles who commit sexual assaults are at high risk of committing other crimes once they reach adulthood but that these crimes are not necessarily sexual. In studies in high schools in 1996, Ryan and others found that 60 percent of the boys stated that it was acceptable for a boy to force sex on a girl. This may explain the high percentage of forced sex seen among high school students surveyed by the Youth Risk Behavior System survey.

The consequences of sexual violence and rape

Victims of rape and sexual assault are at risk for a variety of physical, psychological, and social problems following the rape. Among the long-lasting physical symptoms and illnesses associated with sexual violence are chronic pelvic pain, premenstrual syndrome, gastrointestinal disorders, and a variety of chronic pain disorders, including headache, back pain, and facial pain. Also, between 4 percent and 30 percent of rape victims contract sexually transmitted diseases, including HIV. Unwanted pregnancies arising from rape are another consequence faced by many women. In a study in 2000, researchers Stewart and Trussell estimated that there were 25,000 pregnancies resulting from the 333,000 sexual assaults and rapes reported in the United States in 1998, and that 22,000 of those pregnancies could have been prevented with prompt medical care that included emergency contraception treatment.

Victims of sexual violence exhibit psychological symptoms that are similar to those of victims of other types of trauma, such as war and natural disaster. Some develop post-traumatic stress disorder, which is characterized by emotional detachment, sleep disturbances, and flashbacks. Approximately one-third of rape victims have symptoms that continue for three months or become chronic, or ongoing. Long-term psychological effects experienced by rape victims include anxiety, guilt, nervousness, phobias (irrational fears), substance abuse, sleep disturbances, depression, alienation, and sexual dysfunction. They often distrust others and, according to numerous studies, replay the assault in their minds, putting them at increased risk of being victimized a second time. Depression is also a particular risk for women who have been raped, and women who have been sexually assaulted are more likely to attempt or commit suicide than other women.

ARE RAPISTS THAT WAY FOR LIFE?

Many people believe that sexual offenders or rapists cannot ever be trusted to reform. They believe that if a rapist is released from prison it is only a matter of time before he rapes someone else. This belief is particularly strong in regard to **pedophiles**, or those who sexually molest small children.

Although many sexual offenders do go on to commit new crimes, many do not. In one study in Canada in 1996, Motiuk and Brown found that three and one-half years after release from prison, about one-third of the sex offenders had been convicted of a new criminal offense. About 20 percent of these convictions were for a violent crime, but fewer than 10 percent were for a new sexual offense. The original crime did make a difference—rapists were more likely to commit new violent and sexual crimes than were those convicted of incest. Pedophiles also had a higher recidivism rate, being more likely to return to crime. Those who were younger at the time of release had received a federal (Canadian) prison term for sexual crimes in the past, and those who abused drugs as adults were most likely to commit new sexual offenses.

A DOJ survey in 2003 of about 9,600 released sex offenders in the United States also showed that they were relatively unlikely to commit future sexual assaults. Only about 5 percent of the offenders were rearrested for sex crimes. As in the Canadian study, the younger the offender was at release, the greater the likelihood of rearrest. In addition, receiving little or no counseling or rehabilitation in prison made a sex offender more likely to commit new crimes.

VIOLENCE TOWARD SPECIAL POPULATIONS

Certain populations may have specific concerns, in addition to those faced by anyone who is the victim of a sexual assault. Some of these special populations include teenagers, lesbians, immigrants—especially those who are undocumented or have limited English language skills— men, prisoners, those in the military, the disabled, or the hearing impaired.

One of the groups for which statistics exist is men. Most of us think only women are raped, but this is not true. According to the FBI, one in five men will be raped or sexually assaulted in their lifetime. Most of these will be heterosexual males committing assaults on other heterosexual men. Unlike women, according to the DOJ, males are much more likely to be the victims of violence inflicted by strangers than by family members or other close associates.

See also: Children and Rape; Date Rape; Drugs, Alcohol, and Rape; Gang Rape; Rape Within Abusive Relationships; Sexual Abuse in Institutions; Victims of Rape: Female; Victims of Rape: Male

FURTHER READING

Holmes, Stephen, and Ronald Holmes. *Sex Crimes: Patterns and Behavior.* Thousand Oaks, Calif.: Sage Publications, 2008.

■ RAPE WITHIN ABUSIVE RELATIONSHIPS

Sexual assault can occur within abusive relationships—those that are aggressive, controlling, or violent. Acquaintances, friends, and relatives commit sexual assaults—including rape, child molestation, **incest** (sex between family members who are not husband and wife), and sexual harassment. "Non-strangers" (people we know) commit these crimes more often than strangers. Rape by people victims know can be particularly devastating because the victims are betrayed by a person they cared about and whom they thought cared about them.

PARTNER ABUSE

Partner abuse is aggressive or controlling behavior toward an intimate partner in order to exert power over the partner's actions. The abuse may be physical, sexual, or psychological and emotional. Some of the terms used to describe intimate partner violence include **domestic violence, spousal abuse, battering,** date rape, and **marital rape.**

DID YOU KNOW?

Attacker's Relationship to Victim

(Percent of total attacks of people age 12 and older. Includes rape, attempted rape, and sexual assault)

	1993	1994	1995	1996	1997	1998	1999	2000	2001	2003	2005
All Non-Stranger	72.4%	64.0%	69.8%	67.5%	68.1%	74.0%	69.0%	62.0%	66.0%	70.0%	73.0%
-intimate	10.5%	8.3%	7.0%	7.5%	3.8%	18.0%	20.0%	17.0%	16.0%	12.0%*	28.0%
-other relative	3.2%	2.3%	4.0%	9.2%	6.4%	8.0%	3.0%*	2.0%	2.0%*	8.0%*	7.0%*
-friend/acquaintance	58.7%	53.4%	58.8%	50.8%	58.0%	48.0%	46.0%	43.0%	48.0%	50.0%	38.0%
Stranger	24.4%	30.9%	30.2%	32.4%	31.9%	25.0%	30.0%	34.0%	30.0%	30.0%	26.0%
Unknown	3.2%	4.9%	0.0%	0.0%	0.0%	2.0%	1.0%	4.0%*	4.0%*	0.0%*	2.0%*

*Based on 10 or fewer cases

Sources: Rape, Abuse and Incest National Network (RAINN), 2002; NCVS, 2003 and 2005.

Women are more likely to be abused by a partner than men. The National Violence Against Women Survey found that 25 percent of the women it surveyed had been raped or physically assaulted by an intimate partner at some time in their lives. Only 8 percent of the men surveyed reported such an experience. Intimate partner violence is also more deadly for women. Data collected by the FBI shows that although the number of men killed by intimate partners declined 75 percent from 1976 to 2005, the number of women killed by intimate partners remained steady through 1993, according to the Bureau of Justice Statistics Homicide Trends. Even once the numbers began to drop, the percentage of female homicide victims killed by an intimate partner remained basically the same, about 30 percent.

Fact Or Fiction?

If you are married, your spouse is supposed to be available to you for sexual activity whenever you want it. Therefore, you cannot rape a spouse.

The Facts: Laws of the past 30 years now define marital rape as a crime. Today, no one can legally be forced to have sex. If a partner is forced to have sex, he or she has been raped, even if the perpetrator is a spouse.

Sexual abuse tends to be common in relationships characterized by a pattern of coercive control and increasing entrapment. Single, separated, or divorced women are more likely to be abused by a partner than other women. Other risk factors include pregnancy, age (young people are more likely to be at risk than adults), and alcohol and substance abuse.

Q & A

Question: I like to drink at parties. My sister says if I drink, I am more likely to be raped. Is this true?

Answer: There is a link between substance abuse and sexual assault. Drinking can loosen one's inhibitions. Someone who has consumed alcohol may be more likely to do things that he or she normally would avoid. Drinking may also bring out sexually aggressive behavior in some people. Teens who drink may find themselves in situations where it is hard to use good judgment, be cautious, or protect themselves.

Some people feel that being raped or sexually assaulted by a partner does not have the same impact as being raped by a stranger. Study after study indicates that this idea is false. Those abused by a partner suffer **post-traumatic stress disorder** and **rape trauma syndrome** at the same rates as other rape victims. Like others who suffer from the two syndromes, victims of partner abuse experience shock, memory loss, nightmares, reliving the incident(s) over and over, helplessness, anxiety, and depression. In fact, women raped within the context of an intimate relationship may suffer more severe effects. Psychologists often attribute the severity of the effects to the bond between the victim and the perpetrator; unlike a victim of stranger rape, a person who is raped by an intimate partner feels betrayed. Many also feel a loyalty to their attacker and are therefore more likely to suffer continued and repeated abuse.

Those who are sexually abused by a partner may feel as if they are somehow responsible for the attack. They sometimes feel that if they had been a better person, they would not have been mistreated. Long-term effects of partner abuse often include an inability to trust the opposite sex, a lack of comfort with sex or intimacy, and fear of being assaulted again, even if they no longer live with or see the attacker. Counseling may help individuals confront some of these feelings and heal faster.

CHILD ABUSE

Child sexual abuse can take place within the family (abuse by a parent, stepparent, sibling, or other relative) or outside the home (abuse by a friend, neighbor, babysitter, teacher, or stranger). According to the Department of Justice, the median age of the victims of prisoners convicted of child abuse was younger than 13 years of age—that is, half the victims were older than 13 and half were younger. Those convicted of sex crimes against children tend to be older than those convicted of sex crimes against adults. Nearly 25 percent of child sexual abusers were over age 40; only 10 percent of those who victimized adults were over the age of 40.

Convicted perpetrators of sexual assaults serving time in state prisons report that two-thirds of their victims were under the age of 18, and 58 percent were 12 years of age or younger. In 90 percent of the rapes of children under the age of 12, the child knew the offender, according to police-recorded incident data.

According to the American Academy of Child and Adolescent Psychiatry although there were more than 78,000 cases of child sexual abuse reported in the United States in 2006, children who are sexually abused often do not tell anyone about their abuse. They may fear that disclosure will bring consequences even worse than being victimized again. They may fear not being believed or being blamed by other family members, they may feel guilty if the perpetrator is punished, or they may fear subsequent retaliatory actions by their attacker.

Sexually abused children often have a pronounced inability to trust others. They may feel that something is wrong with them or that the abuse is somehow their fault. Many feel guilty, not only about the sexual activity, but also about being different from their peers. They may experience anger toward their parents or guardians and feel disloyal or fearful of bringing disruption to the family. An abuser may threaten the child with a loss of love or with violence if he or she tells. It is important to identify victims of sexual abuse early. With early detection, the child can receive the help he or she needs for appropriate psychological development and healthy adult functioning.

DATE OR ACQUAINTANCE RAPE

Date rape (also referred to as acquaintance rape and hidden rape) is increasingly viewed as a serious problem, particularly on college campuses. Many victims of date rape are unsure if their experience was really a sexual assault, because they knew the perpetrator and went willingly with him or her.

The perpetrator of acquaintance rape is almost always a man. Although both men and women can be raped, women are most often the targets of this violence. It is particularly difficult to collect accurate statistics of the number of acquaintance rapes, as the victims are among the least likely to report a sexual assault.

The following warning signs might indicate the possibility of abusive behavior in the future:

- Acts emotionally abusive and frequently insults his or her partner, makes belittling comments in front of others, ignores partner, or acts angry when his or her partner initiates an action or idea
- Tells partner with whom he or she may be friends, how he or she should dress, or tries to control other elements of partner's life
- Talks negatively about women in general
- Becomes jealous for no reason
- Drinks heavily, uses drugs, or tries to get partner drunk
- Gets angry if partner does not want to get drunk, high, have sex, or go with him or her to an isolated place
- Is physically violent to partner or others
- Acts in an intimidating way by invading partner's "personal space" (sits too close, speaks as if he or she knows partner much better than he or she does, touches partner after being told not to)
- Is unable to handle sexual and emotional frustrations without becoming angry

Be careful when getting to know someone if he or she exhibits some or all of these warning signs. These warning signs should cause a person to reconsider the relationship and choose not to continue.

Date rape is controversial because of a lack of agreement about the definition of consent. It may be unrealistic to ask a sexual partner for consent to each subsequent step in sexual intimacy. However, doing so is the only way to be sure that a partner agrees to go further. Anytime a person says "stop," his or her partner should stop immediately. To continue is rape. Just because someone has agreed to sexual relations with his or her partner in the past does not mean that the person owes his or her partner sex in the future. Acquaintance rape is often violent and is no less an assault than a rape perpetrated by a stranger. One of the ways that the courts have recognized this fact is by making marital rape illegal in all 50 states.

See also: Date Rape; Female Rights; Male Role in Rape; Rape and Society; Sexual Assault, Types of

■ SAFE AREAS, ESTABLISHING

Establishing safe areas involves creating places where people can live as free as possible from rape, other sexual assaults, and violence. Among the places that can be made safer are homes, schools, and communities.

Rape prevention measures, both proactive and reactive, are important for keeping people safe from rape and other forms of sexual assault. Once individuals learn how they can protect themselves in a sometimes-unsafe world, they may wonder if there is anything that can be done to make their home, school, or community a safer place. The answer is yes. Many people of all ages, including high school students, are working toward this goal.

SAFETY AT HOME

According to the 2005 National Crime Victimization Survey, 60 percent of all rapes occur in or near the home. Therefore, it makes sense to do whatever is necessary to make one's home a safe haven.

The most important aspect of keeping a family safe from rape, other sexual assaults, and violence is communication among people living in a household. When household members communicate and cooperate in creating and implementing prevention guidelines and strategies, the entire family can live more safely. If some family members are unwilling to cooperate, individuals can still formulate a safety plan with those who are willing to take a stand.

Ways to protect your family at home

To make your family safer, experts suggest the following:

- Make your home more physically secure by adding dead-bolt locks to all doors and windows and adding lights to all entries and pathways. Pull down the shades at night.

- Keep track of where family members are going when they go out and approximately when they will return.

IF SEXUAL ABUSE OR DOMESTIC VIOLENCE IS A PROBLEM

Anyone who is being sexually abused at home can secure help even if he or she feels the situation is hopeless. If one cannot confide in a close friend, relative, or another trusted person, he or she can make an anonymous phone call to a rape crisis or domestic violence hot-line. Such a call can provide a safe, secure first step. The people who answer the phones are knowledgeable about sexual abuse, sexual assault, and rape. They are trained to provide information and options that can make a difference. No one has to suffer from abuse.

Whenever a family member becomes a victim of sexual abuse or assault, the problem seriously affects everyone in the family. It is important to find someone to talk to who can help, and once again, a hotline is an excellent place to start. The Hotlines and Help Sites section at the back of this book provides a list of helpful national sites.

SAFETY AT SCHOOL

When most people think about violence in school, they often think about bullying, physical assaults, and gun violence. Yet, the U.S. Department of Education reported that an estimated 5,000 rapes or acts of sexual assault occurred in the nation's public schools during the 2005–6 school year. The U.S. Department of Justice's Bureau of Justice Statistics reported that students were the victims of more than 59,000 serious violent crimes at school, including rape and sexual assault during school year 2005–6. There were also almost 1.5 million violent incidents, some of which were also rapes and sexual assaults.

It is important to report violence that happens at school. According to the National Center for Education Statistics in 2002, more than 88 percent of all students surveyed who were victimized at school never reported the incident. If school officials do not know that a student has been harmed, they cannot address problems.

Any student who is threatened with sexual assault or is being harassed or bullied should inform a trusted teacher, a guidance counselor, the principal, or another school official. Those who are reluctant to report a problem alone can ask a friend to come along. If students are worried that others will find out that they spoke to school authorities, they should share that concern with the staff. They can also contact Safe School Helpline (1-800-418-6423, extension 359), a national hotline that more than 4,000 schools encourage their students to use. Safe School Helpline gives students a way to anonymously report school violence. After collecting information from students' phone calls, the staff passes that information on to school authorities. The identity of the caller remains unknown throughout the entire process.

Fact Or Fiction?

Boys are less likely than girls to report that they have been the victim of a violent crime at school because boys do not want anyone to know that they cannot handle a problem.

The Facts: According to "The Condition of Education," a report published in 2003 by the National Center for Education Statistics, boys are more likely than girls to tell school authorities that they have been victimized.

Tips on staying safe at school

Danger zones in schools are areas where there are few or no people. Students should avoid lingering in those places—particularly in stairways, empty classrooms, restrooms, or unlit areas before and after school hours.

Experts also suggest that students avoid staying after school alone. If a student is participating in a sport or other after-school activity, he or she should plan to leave with a friend. If it is necessary to meet with a teacher after school, students should exit by the most traveled stairway or hallway. They should also avoid using a restroom after school unless other people are also using it.

Q & A

Question: A group of boys at my school have said they're going to rape me, and I'm afraid they will do it. My friend and I told the principal about it, but nothing he has done has helped. What can I do?

Answer: School administrators are responsible for ensuring the safety of every student in the school. Have you returned to the principal to tell him that you are still being threatened? If you have and nothing is being done, ask your parents for help. They may need to talk to the principal or speak to the superintendent or another administrator who is in charge of the entire school system. If that does not help, your parents may need to discuss the matter with the police. As your safety is important, you have the right to demand protection.

Students taking a stand against violence

Some students in high schools throughout the country have formed organizations to make their schools safer places. They want to stop all violence at school.

Students Against Violence Everywhere (SAVE) is a national organization based in Raleigh, North Carolina. The group works with young people to improve school safety. Students who form SAVE chapters in their schools have organized crime prevention fairs, in which police officers and other law enforcement specialists offer information about preventing crime. Other SAVE groups have improved and beautified school property in hopes that their efforts will inspire other students to care for the school environment. As part of yet another popular SAVE project, students identify areas in the school where conflicts and violence occur. SAVE members then share the list with school officials and ask for their cooperation in finding ways to improve those areas.

TEENS SPEAK

When I First Arrived at a Large High School, I Was Overwhelmed: There Were Many Things That Upset Me

I'm a senior at a large high school. When I first arrived in the ninth grade, I was overwhelmed. I liked my teachers, and I had my friends from middle school, but there were things that upset me. For one thing, there were many fights on the school grounds, in the halls, and even in the classrooms before class. There were other kinds of violence too.

When I was in the 10th grade, a boy in my history class cornered me in a stairway. He pushed me up against the wall and thrust his pelvis into me. He told me he would track me down and have sex with me under the bleachers after my basketball practice. I told my teacher about it and he never came near me again. But I was scared all the time.

I got so sick of being scared that I joined a group at school that's working to make our school a more peaceful place. We did a survey and it showed that 92 percent of the kids in my school didn't want fights and other violence.

The year I joined we organized a peace festival that lasted an entire week. Every day that week at lunch, we had speakers who talked about their favorite sport or hobby. One man brought a small kayak and talked about paddling white-water rapids; a woman demonstrated calligraphy; and an older man executed some karate moves. During that week, there weren't any fights in the cafeteria. In the weeks after the festival, we organized after-school events where kids could come and practice calligraphy and learn a little karate.

Maybe the events we planned didn't stop the violence, but it encouraged people to make their lives better, and I think that's a good first step. Over the last three years we've done a lot of projects, and I believe we've made a difference. At least I know a lot of kids who are involved feel better about school.

SAFETY IN THE COMMUNITY

In many communities, people in all walks of life are joining forces to keep themselves, their families, and their neighbors safe from violent crime. The first priority of most of these community coalitions is education. To stop rape and other violent crimes, concerned citizens have organized violence and rape prevention courses and workshops, including programs for young people who are most at risk of being the victims of a violent crime.

Many community groups support rape crisis centers. They also fund and help build youth centers, where young people can gather for fun but safe activities after school and on weekends. Other groups help find employment for teens and adults in the community because they know that high unemployment is often associated with increases in the rate of violence in a community.

A national program called Teens, Crime, and the Community (TCC) has inspired more than 1 million teenagers to participate in projects to help make their community safer. A TCC program called the Youth Safety Corps (YSC) involves young people in crime prevention activities. Students work with community volunteers to identify safety issues that face teens in both school and the community. Then YSC groups develop and carry out projects that address those issues. In some communities, students have painted murals over walls covered with hate language. Some have organized programs for middle school students to teach them how to be safe from violent crime, deal with bullying, and resist peer pressure when offered alcohol and drugs. Teens have also worked with community leaders to develop plans for youth centers.

Although these projects never eliminate violence completely, they do teach individuals how to be a little safer from violence. These efforts also have another important effect; they help people feel good about themselves and their community. People who participate in civic projects often feel that they are playing an important role in making their community a healthier and more peaceful place to live and work.

See also: Educating the Community; Help and Support; Prevention of Rape: Being Proactive; Prevention of Rape: Being Reactive

FURTHER READING

Denny, Todd. *Unexpected Allies: Men Who Stop Rape.* Victoria, B.C.: Trafford Publishing, 2007.

Feuereisen, Patti. *Invisible Girls: The Truth About Sexual Abuse A Book for Teen Girls, Young Women, and Everyone Who Cares About Them.* New York: Seal Press, 2005.

Rutledge, Jill Zimmerman. *Dealing with the Stuff That Makes Life Tough: The Ten Things That Stress Teen Girls Out and How to Cope with Them.* New York: McGraw-Hill, 2003.

Wells, Donna Koren, and Bruce C. Morris. *Keep Safe! 101 Ways to Enhance Your Safety and Protect Your Family.* Alameda, CA: Hunter House, 2003.

■ SEXUAL ABUSE IN INSTITUTIONS

Sexual assaults that take place in institutions such as group homes, prisons, juvenile detention facilities, nursing homes, mental hospitals, schools, and colleges. People who are in institutions tend to be vulnerable to abuse because they are often unable to protect themselves. They are under the care of others—a charitable foundation, government or religious group, or other organization.

RAPE IN MENTAL INSTITUTIONS

Although statistics on the frequency of rapes in mental institutions are not available, national studies suggest that women inmates who are raped are unlikely to be believed if they report an assault. These studies also show that abuse occurs in expensive facilities as well as those that primarily serve low-income patients. Often rapes that occur in large mental hospitals are handled internally and are not reported to the police.

Although other patients are most often responsible for rapes in mental hospitals, staff members are sometimes the perpetrators. Background checks of previous criminal activity are usually performed before someone is hired, but checks do not catch everyone who might be a danger to those in his or her care.

RAPE IN PRISONS

Although inmates often enter prisons or detention centers with a history of abuse, rape is also common in prisons and juvenile detention facilities. Most rapes are between prisoners, although guards and other staff members are sometimes the perpetrators. According to a 2007 report from the Bureau of Justice Statistics, 4.5 percent of prison inmates reported being the victim of a sexual assault. This suggests that more than 60,000 of the nation's approximately 2 million prisoners are raped each year.

Prisoners may also be coerced into trading sex for favorable treatment or for goods, such as food or cigarettes. First-time offenders and prisoners still in their teens are the most likely to be sexually assaulted. Prisoners who have been raped are also at risk for sexually transmitted diseases (STDs) because they have no way of protecting themselves. Women who are sexually assaulted in jail are additionally at risk for unwanted pregnancies.

DID YOU KNOW?

Sexual Violence in Juvenile Facilities

Of the more than 4,000 allegations of sexual misconduct reported for juvenile justice facilities in 2005 and 2006, approximately half of the complaints were for youth-on-youth violence and half were for sexual violence or harassment by facility staff. Of the substantiated complaints, 40 percent were perpetrated by staff.

Source: Bureau of Justice Statistics, 2008.

In 2003, Congress passed the Prison Rape Elimination Act, the first federal law to deal with sexual assaults behind bars. The act requires that the government gather statistics about the problem, develop guidelines for states, create a review panel to hold annual hearings, and offer state grants to combat the problem. The law also sets standards for investigating and eliminating rape and holds the states accountable if they fail to do so. It requires that corrections officials provide a confidential way for inmates to report rapes and provides incentives to state and local governments to prevent and punish rapes in prisons.

Fact Or Fiction?

Those who commit crimes take the risk that they will be raped in prison.

The Facts: Being a convicted criminal does not mean that one deserves to be raped. Federal law requires that prisons have methods in place so that rape and other sexual assaults can be reported confidentially. However, only the victim can decide if the facility in which he or she is housed can be trusted.

Rape in prison is against the law. The U.S. Supreme Court has held that prisoner rape is a violation of the Eighth Amendment to the U.S. Constitution (prohibiting cruel and unusual punishment). Inmates who rape can be tried for sexual assault and, if convicted, sentenced to additional time in jail. However, prisons often handle assaults internally, and most prison rapists are never brought to trial.

RAPE IN JUVENILE DETENTION FACILITIES

According to a 2000 study by the Office of Juvenile Justice and Delinquency Prevention, approximately 107,000 youths in the United States are incarcerated on any given day. Of these, approximately 14,500 are housed in adult facilities. The rest are located in juvenile detention facilities. In 2003, 96,665 juveniles were held in residential placement facilities, either private, state, or local. The Coalition for Juvenile Justice estimates that 33 percent of the juveniles in detention facilities are there for violent offenses such as assault, rape, or murder, and robbery.

DID YOU KNOW?

History of Abuse Before Admission to Prison

Before admission	State Inmates		Federal Inmates		Jail Inmates		Probationists	
	Male	Female	Male	Female	Male	Female	Male	Female
Ever abused	16.1%	57.2%	7.2%	39.9%	12.9%	47.6%	9.3%	40.4%
Physically[a]	13.4	46.5	6.0	32.3	10.7	37.3	7.4	33.5
Sexually[b]	5.8	39.0	2.2	22.8	5.6	37.2	4.1	25.2
Both	3.0	28.0	1.1	15.1	3.3	26.9	2.1	18.3
Age of victim at time of abuse								
17 or younger	14.4%	36.7%	5.8%	23.0%	11.9%	36.6%	8.8%	28.2%
18 or older	4.3	45.0	2.7	31.0	2.3	26.7	1.1	24.7
Both	2.5	24.7	1.3	14.2	1.3	15.8	0.5	12.5
Age of abuser								
Adult	15.0%	55.8%	6.9%	39.0%	12.1%	46.0%	8.5%	39.2%
Juvenile only	0.9	1.0	0.2	0.3	0.8	1.3	0.6	1.2

[a] Includes those both physically and sexually abused

[b] Includes those abused in both age categories

Source: Department of Justice, 2008.

Although youths incarcerated in adult prisons are up to five times more likely to be raped than those housed in juvenile detention facilities, it does not mean that rape does not occur in the juvenile facilities. In 2004, there were 2,821 alleged incidents of sexual violence reported in juvenile facilities, 41 percent of which involved accusations against staff. A 2000 study by the Juvenile Forensic Evaluation Resource Center reports that "the daily reality of juveniles confined in many 'treatment' facilities is one of violence, predatory behavior, and punitive incarceration." Although there are few, if any, estimates of the level of rape in juvenile detention facilities, the Prison Rape Elimination Act, passed in 2003, allows for future surveys to help determine this information.

RAPE IN NURSING HOMES

People who reside in nursing homes are particularly vulnerable to sexual abuse by other residents or staff members. A study by A Perfect Cause, a nonprofit disability and elder rights group, showed that hundreds of registered sex offenders live in nursing homes. About 44 percent of these offenders are under 60 years of age, dispelling the notion that sex offenders are only placed in nursing homes when they are too old to pose a risk. Families have a difficult time getting information about sex offenders prior to placing a family member in a home. Many homes also fail to promptly report alleged physical and sexual abuse of residents, and few cases are prosecuted, particularly if the assailant is another resident.

Q & A

Question: My grandmother is ill and needs to go into a nursing home. Is there any way for my family to find out if any registered sex offenders are residing in the home?

Answer: A Perfect Cause, the nonprofit disability and elders' rights advocacy group, maintains a database of sex offenders who reside in nursing homes on its Web site at http://www.aperfectcause. org. Individuals can search by the name of the nursing home or the offender. Similar information may be available from a state agency that registers nursing homes.

Although federal regulations prohibit nursing facilities from employing anyone who has been convicted of resident abuse, federal laws do not specifically require a criminal background check of employees. Although many states do require such checks, they may not be required for all employees or only cover individuals who have been convicted of crimes in settings other than a nursing home. To complicate matters, background checks are not always completed before the person begins work. Furthermore, state criminal background checks typically cover only one state, so convictions in other states are often missed.

See also: Law and Rape, The; Rape Statistics; Safe Areas, Establishing; Sexual Violence and Children; Victims of Rape: Female; Victims of Rape: Male

■ SEXUAL ASSAULT, TYPES OF

Sexual assault is a broader term than rape. In addition to what we traditionally consider rape, it refers to other types of unwanted sexual touching or penetration without consent, including

- Forced **sodomy** (anal intercourse)
- Forced oral sex (oral-genital contact)
- Rape by other body parts (including a finger)
- Rape by a foreign object
- **Sexual battery** (the unwanted touching of another person for the purpose of sexual arousal)

Sexual assault can be verbal, visual, or anything that forces a person to join in unwanted sexual contact or attention. It can include **voyeurism** (when someone watches private sexual acts); **exhibitionism** (when someone exposes himself or herself in public); incest (sexual contact between family members who are not husband and wife); and sexual harassment. Such assaults can occur in an isolated place, on a date, or even in the home.

RAPE

The legal definition of rape varies from state to state. However, rape is generally defined as forced or **nonconsensual** sexual intercourse.

Although in the past the legal term *rape* traditionally referred to forced vaginal penetration of a woman by a male assailant, in most places the statutes, or laws, are now gender-neutral. Rape may be accomplished by fear, threats of harm, or actual physical force. Rape may also include situations in which penetration is accomplished when the victim is unable to give consent or is prevented from resisting, due to being intoxicated, drugged, unconscious, or asleep.

TEENS SPEAK

I Didn't Know It Was Rape

When I was 16, I went on a date with a guy I had met at a party. I didn't know him well, but I figured since I had met him at a friend's house it would be okay. For a long time afterward I wouldn't use the word "rape" to describe what happened to me, even though he held me down and forced me to have sex with him. I thought that if I willingly went out with him and drove around in his car, that this couldn't be rape. I thought only strangers could rape you. It wasn't until my teacher was talking about date rape in health class that I realized that I had been raped. I know it sounds stupid, but I really didn't think I was raped before that.

Date rape

Date or acquaintance rape refers to those sexual assaults committed by someone you know, such as a date, teacher, employer, or family member. Date rape, which is a specific type of acquaintance rape, generally refers to forced or unwanted sexual activity that occurs within a dating relationship. Date rape remains a particular problem on college campuses.

Marital rape

Prior to the 1970s, most people did not consider forced sex within a marriage to be rape. Today, however, the legal systems in all 50 states recognize that forced and unwanted sexual intercourse is rape, even within the context of marriage (though some states have exceptions). Still, even with the changes in the law, there are individuals who question whether marital rape should really be a crime. A 2008 study examining attitudes about marital rape found that unfortunately many people still do not consider it to be as serious an offense as other types of acquaintance rape. According to a 1990 study, researchers Russell and associates estimated that between 10 and 14 percent of married women experience rape in marriage. Similar problems with forced intercourse are sometimes found in other intimate partnerships, such as those of **cohabitating** couples, or couples who live together but are not legally married, and gay or lesbian couples.

Incest
Incest generally refers to situations where the perpetrator is related to the victim. Traditionally, incest referred to sexual intercourse among family members (other than husband and wife), or those legally barred from marriage. However, most consider sexual activity between stepparents or other parental figures in the home and their stepchildren, or between step-siblings, also to be incest.

Statutory rape
Statutory rape refers to sexual intercourse with a child or teen under a specified age (usually 18 years old). Statutory rape is another example of sexual assault. All 50 states and the District of Columbia have laws criminalizing statutory rape. Such laws typically base the severity of the crime on the age of the minor and the age difference between the minor and her or his assailant. The age at which an adolescent may consent to sexual intercourse varies by state and ranges from 14 to 18 years of age. The consent of someone younger than the **age of consent** is legally irrelevant because the individual is defined as being incapable of consenting. In other words, it does not matter if the minor consents to sex or not; in all cases, sex with a minor is considered rape.

Drug-facilitated rape
"Drug-facilitated sexual assault" is generally used to describe situations in which victims are subjected to **nonconsensual** sexual acts while they are incapacitated or unconscious because of the effects of alcohol and/or other drugs and, therefore, prevented from resisting or giving consent. The most common drugs given clandestinely to

victims are Rohypnol or GHB, although there also are many others. These drugs, when slipped into someone's drink, can render the person unconscious or so out of it that he or she is unable to resist the sexual advances of the assailant. Never leave your drink unattended if you are in a bar or at a party, and if you start to feel drunker than you would have expected from the amount of alcohol you have consumed, ask a trusted friend to take you home immediately.

If someone is raped and suspects he or she has been drugged, it is important to have a urine test as part of the medical treatment following the assault. The drugs commonly used to facilitate rape show up more easily in urine than they do in blood. Prosecuting the rapist is much more difficult without this crucial physical evidence.

Rape with an object
When someone forcibly places an object in another person's vagina or anus, this is a sexual assault. The perpetrator can be prosecuted for rape, and the victim should report the crime as he or she would report any other rape. The victim should also seek medical treatment following the assault.

Sodomy
Sodomy is usually defined legally as oral or anal sex between two people. Until recently, sodomy was illegal in many states, even when it took place between mutually consenting adults in the privacy of their own homes. These laws, which were highly discriminatory against gays and lesbians, were overturned in 2003 with a Supreme Court decision that stated individuals were entitled to respect in their private lives. Now sodomy is only illegal if it is forced, or nonconsensual. If someone is forced to engage in oral or anal sex against his or her will, this is a crime, even if the person is not a victim of vaginal penetration.

VOYEURISM
Voyeurism refers to the act of becoming sexually aroused by looking at unsuspecting individuals who may be naked, in the process of removing their clothing, or participating in sexual activity. Some, but not all, voyeurs masturbate during, or shortly after, their voyeuristic activities. If those being observed are unaware or do not consent to being watched, then voyeurism is a crime. According to Psych-Net, voyeurs typically begin their activities before the age of 15. The

Types of Sexual Crimes

Sexual Crimes	Types	Definition
Rape		Sexual penetration without the individual's consent, obtained by force or threat of physical harm, or when the victim is unable to give consent
	Acquaintance rape	Sexual assault committed by someone known to the victim
	Date rape	A type of acquaintance rape; sexual assault perpetrated in the context of a dating relationship
	Drug-facilitated rape	Sexual assault perpetrated on a victim who has been rendered unconscious or incapacitated by the use of alcohol or drugs and who is therefore unable to consent to sexual activity
	Incest	Nonconsensual sexual activity between family members who are not husband and wife
	Marital rape	Nonconsensual sexual activity between married partners
	Sodomy	Nonconsensual oral or anal sex
	Statutory rape	Sexual activity between someone at or over the age of consent with someone below the age of consent
Voyeurism		Observation of non-consenting individuals in acts of disrobing or sexual activity
Exhibitionism		Exposure of the genitals to non-consenting individuals
Child abuse (sexual)		Any sexual act involving a child that involves force, threat, or manipulation; child sexual abuse may be committed by adults or by other children

individual may become so invested in the voyeuristic activity that it becomes his or her sole sexual behavior. Voyeurs are sometimes known as Peeping Toms. Note that some types of voyeurism are legal and relatively common in our society, such as adults downloading Internet pornography, watching X-rated movies, or reading pornographic magazines.

EXHIBITIONISM

Exhibitionists become sexually aroused by exposing their genitals to others. Usually, a key factor in the exhibitionist's arousal is that the victim be a stranger or someone unsuspecting of the upcoming event. Exhibitionism most often involves non-consenting persons. Sometimes the exhibitionist masturbates while exposing himself or herself but, in general, exhibitionists make no further attempt at sexual contact with the stranger. An exhibitionist, who is sexually aroused by the shock or surprise of the victim, is not seeking physical contact and will not usually commit rape, although some rapists may show signs of exhibitionism as well. However, exhibitionist behavior can still be a crime.

CHILD ABUSE AND SEXUAL ASSAULT

Most states also define any sexual assault occurring in childhood as child abuse. The National Center on Child Abuse and Neglect defines childhood sexual abuse as "contact or interaction between a child and an adult when the child is being used for the sexual stimulation of that adult or another person." Childhood sexual abuse may be committed by another minor when that person is either significantly older than the victim (more than five years) or when the abuser is in a position of power or control over the child.

Q & A

Question: I keep asking this girl out, and she keeps saying no. I really like her a lot, and I want to go out with her. I think she just says no hoping I'll ask her again. How can I convince her to go out with me?

Answer: If you think you are flirting with someone, but they do not respond the way you want them to, consider that you might be making them uncomfortable. The bottom line is that if the person receiving your sexual or romantic attention doesn't want it and you continue, that's harassment and you should stop. Some ways to tell if you might be harassing someone include if the person does not seem happy with your attention, if you flirt but they do not flirt back, if you make a sexual joke and they do not laugh, or if the person seems to be avoiding you.

SEXUAL HARASSMENT

Sexual harassment is defined as any unwelcome sexual attention—whether it is unwanted sexual advances, requests for sexual favors, sexual jokes, or similar behaviors that interfere with a person's ability to function in school or at work. Although the person committing the harassment may intend to make his or her victim feel good with the unwanted attention, any sexual attention that makes a person feel uncomfortable can be considered harassment. Sexual harassment is not only committed by men against women. Both men and women can sexually harass individuals of the same or opposite gender, and harassment can be committed by a person of any age. Same-sex sexual harassment may be more difficult for an individual to admit to—and more difficult to prosecute—but that does not mean it does not happen.

Fact Or Fiction?

It is okay for my teacher to flirt with me.

The Facts: It is never okay for an adult to flirt with a teenager, especially in a situation where the adult has some power over the teen, like a teacher has over a student. This is true whether the teacher is a man or a woman and whether you are a boy or a girl. If the teacher persists in flirting with you, this could be considered sexual harassment. You should tell someone in charge about his or her behavior, particularly if a teacher continues flirting with you after you tell him or her to stop.

Some flirting between teens (or adults) is normal and healthy, but sometimes it can be hard to tell the difference between flirting and sexual harassment. In general, harmless flirting is wanted and makes the person feel good. Sexual harassment, on the other hand, is unwanted, one-sided, makes the victim feel put down or ugly, power-less, bad, or dirty. This unwelcome attention is a violation of the rules in both schools and workplaces and is also against the law.

See also: Abusive Sexual Behavior; Children and Rape; Date Rape; Gang Rape; Law and Rape, The; Rape Kits and Evidence Collection; Rape Within Abusive Relationships; Sexual Harassment; Sexual Violence and Children; Statutory Rape

FURTHER READING
Aranow, Vicki. *Journey to Wholeness: Healing from the Trauma of Rape.* New York: Crown, 2000.
Domitrz, Michael. *May I Kiss You: A Candid Look at Dating, Communication, Respect, and Sexual Assault Awareness.* Oxnard, CA: Awareness Publishing, 2003.

■ SEXUAL HARASSMENT
Sexual harassment is a form of sexual assault that involves unwanted and repeated sexual advances, requests for sexual favors, other ver-bal taunts, and/or physical conduct of an unwelcome sexual nature. Some people regard sexual harassment as a form of bullying with a sexual component. Like other sexual assaults, sexual harassment can cause mental and emotional damage. It can also lead to violence.

The 2000 book *Faces of Violence in Schools*, edited by D. S. Sandhu, offers a broad-based definition of sexual harassment with four key components:

1. Sexual harassment is one-sided and unwelcome.

2. It is about power, not physical attraction.

3. The harassment occurs repeatedly.

4. It does not stop even after a confrontation—the victim simply cannot get the offender to cease his or her harassing behavior.

In 2001, the American Association of University Women con-ducted a survey on sexual harassment in public schools. Entitled *Hostile Hallways*, it questioned 2,063 students in grades eight through 11. The survey found that 83 percent of girls and 79 percent of boys reported experiencing some form of harassment. According to a 2007 report from the Department of Education, conducted during the 2005–6 school year, approximately 3 percent of students reported sexual harassment by their peers. This is a much lower number than found by the 2001 Hostile Hallways survey. This disparity likely reflects the difference between an official department of education report and one in which students were surveyed directly. As with many other types of sexual violence, sexual harassment is typically underreported.

For many students, sexual harassment was an ongoing experience: More than one in four students reported that it occurred repeatedly. This percentage was unaffected by whether the school was urban, suburban, or rural.

About 76 percent of the students described nonphysical forms of harassment, while 58 percent also experienced physical harassment. Nonphysical harassment included taunting, rumors, graffiti, jokes, or sexual gestures. More than 30 percent of all students reported experiencing physical harassment often or occasionally.

For most respondents (76 percent), the people who harassed them were other students. Girls were more likely than boys to experience harassment, 85 percent to 67 percent. Half of the boys reporting harassment had been nonphysically harassed by a single girl or woman and 39 percent by a group of girls or women. Similarly, girls were most likely to report harassment by a boy or man (73 percent in nonphysical harassment; 84 percent in physical harassment). Only 7 percent of boys and girls experiencing physical or nonphysical harassment reported being harassed by a teacher.

Onset of harassment

For more than one-third (35 percent) of the students who reported being harassed, the disturbing treatment began in elementary school. Students also reported that most harassment occurred at school. About 61 percent reported that physical harassment took place in the classroom, while 56 percent reported nonphysical harassment in the classroom. About 71 percent reported physical harassment in the halls, and 64 percent experienced nonphysical harassment in the halls.

Many students admitted that they had committed some form of harassment. Slightly more than half of the respondents (54 percent) said that they had sexually harassed someone at school, a decrease from 1993, when 59 percent admitted as much. In particular, boys were less likely in 1993 to report being a perpetrator than in 2001 (57 percent in 1993 and 66 percent in 2001).

Fact Or Fiction?

People have been saying rude, sexual things to classmates in schoolyards forever. It's not a big deal.

The Facts: Sexual harassment not only makes a person feel bad emotionally, it can actually make someone physically ill. A 2007 article published in the journal *Violence Against Women* found that not only did more than half of high school girls experience sexual harassment, and more than one third experience unwanted sexual advances, but that those experiences also significantly impacted girls' physical and emotional health.

PREVENTING SEXUAL HARASSMENT

The American Association of University Women prepared a guide for students to accompany their *Hostile Hallways* report. The guide suggests using the following strategies to prevent harassment.

- If someone harasses you, tell him or her to stop. If you are uncomfortable confronting the person directly, do it in writing.

- If you are harassed, tell an adult. Be persistent. If the first person you go to does not respond, go to someone else until you are taken seriously.

- Remind yourself that sexual harassment is illegal and must stop. Do not tell yourself (or believe it if anyone else tells you) that it's your fault.

- If you feel scared, uncomfortable, or threatened by the way a date is treating you, tell a trusted friend or adult and get help.

- Keep a journal of your experiences with sexual harassment. It may prove helpful if you need to recall particular details of the harassment.

■ Interrupt any harassment you observe and tell an adult you trust. Don't be a bystander.

Sexual harassment policies are regulated under Title IX, the same legal statute that is used to ensure that there is equal gender access to sports and other school facilities. In 2008, the Department of Education released a pamphlet designed to help curb the problem of sexual harassment in school, in order to address changes in the legal climate that had occurred over time. Titled *Sexual Harassment: It's Not Academic,* the pamphlet focuses both on educating students about what is and what is not sexual harassment and on how individuals should report incidents that occur.

The pamphlet also reminds students that schools are legally obligated to deal with incidents of harassment which have been reported to officials. On the one hand this should help encourage students to bring their problems to the attention of someone in charge so that they can worry about their schoolwork instead of about being harassed. On the other hand, it is also important for students to know that in certain circumstances, schools may not be able to honor requests for victim confidentiality if doing so could make it difficult to confront an aggressor and put other students at risk.

SOCIAL ASSUMPTIONS

As teens establish their sexual identities, their sexuality and the sexuality of others can become a topic of conversation. Many find it difficult to know what kinds of discussions are acceptable for discussion and what kinds are not. As a rule, discussing another person's sexuality with others is not acceptable.

Counselors and others who work with teens suggest that they monitor the way they speak and what they talk about. It is not a good idea to assume that because you find a topic acceptable, others will. A good rule of thumb might be, "Would a reasonable person of the opposite sex find this embarrassing or offensive?" If the answer is "yes," perhaps whatever you have to say would be better left unsaid.

PEOPLE YOU LEAST EXPECT

A 2003 study of sexual harassment in secondary schools published in the research journal *Sex Roles* found that adults at school were responsible for 27 percent of the sexual harassment of students. Teachers made up 81 percent of the offending group. Although most sexual harassment is by students' peers, a 2008 summary report from the National Center for Women and Girls in Education explored the fact that 40 percent of elementary and high school students report that teachers and other school staff harass students in their schools.

Q & A

Question: What's wrong with telling a dirty joke?

Answer: The problem is that a joke is not always a joke. Although you may not mean anything harmful by telling a sexual joke, some individuals may find it uncomfortable, or even offensive, to hear. A 1998 study in the journal *Sex Roles* showed that college students who enjoyed aggressive sexual humor also held sexually aggressive attitudes that could foster rape.

Coaches, teachers, and other adults, including parents, sometimes unthinkingly make remarks about people or express ideas that can be damaging. Some grew up during a time when words and attitudes that are now considered unacceptable were tolerated. Today, those words and attitudes are considered insensitive at best and offensive at worst.

Fortunately, institutional policies and legal boundaries are being established so that people are aware that certain comments, gestures, and actions are not acceptable. In 1998, the University of California, for example, established a system-wide Policy on Sexual Harassment, which states that unwelcome sexual advances, requests for sexual favors, and other verbal or physical conduct of a sexual nature con- stitute sexual harassment. This behavior is prohibited both by the law and by the university, and anyone whose behavior violates this policy may find themselves facing disciplinary measures or a lawsuit.

When in doubt, refrain from making sexual or suggestive advances toward others. The most important guide for determining whether to say something about or to another person is to consider how the other person might feel if he or she heard the remark.

See also: Help and Support; Safe Areas, Establishing; Sexual Abuse in Institutions

■ SEXUAL VIOLENCE AND CHILDREN

Any forced sexual act, unwanted attempt to obtain a sexual act, or unwanted sexual comments or advances, in any setting, with persons under the age of 18 is sexual violence against children. Sexual violence ranges from forced vaginal, anal, or oral penetration to sexual humiliation. According to the Child Maltreatment report from the Department of Health and Human Services Administration for Children and Families, more than 1 million children were victims of abuse in 2006, and 78,000 of them, or almost 10 percent, were victims of sexual abuse.

Although most sexual crimes tend to be underreported, the National Center for Victims of Crime describes child sexual abuse, especially child sexual abuse within families, as one of the least discussed crimes in the nation. The victims often conceal the crime because of guilt, shame, fear, and social and familial pressures.

SEXUAL ASSAULT AND THE AGE OF CONSENT

Every state has laws that seek to protect children who are considered too young to understand what it means to consent to sexual activities. Known as statutory rape laws, these acts prohibit adult-child relationships but vary in their definition of when childhood ends. The legal age of consent is 18 years in 11 states, 17 years in six states, and 16 years in 33 states.

According to a 2000 report from the Bureau of Justice Statistics (BJS), 67 percent of all victims of sexual assault reported to law enforcement agencies were under the age of 18, and 34 percent of all victims were under the age of 12. The study found that females are at greatest risk of sexual assault at the age of 14 and males at the age of four. Even at that age, a male's risk of assault is approximately 50 percent of a female's risk.

In general, the BJS study found that almost 90 percent of all reported victims of sexual assault were female. The proportion of female victims increased with age. About 69 percent of victims under the age of six were female. Females accounted for 73 percent of victims under the age of 12 and 82 percent of the victims under the age of 18.

Q & A

Question: What effect does child sexual abuse have on victims later in life?

Answer: Having a history of sexual abuse as a child puts a woman at risk for additional abuse later in life. According to the 2004 Department of Justice Report *Violence Against Women, Identifying Risk Factors,* individuals who had been sexually abused during childhood and adolescence were almost three times as likely to be sexually abused as adults as those individuals who had never been abused. They were also twice as likely to have experienced any domestic violence.

A history of abuse during childhood may also make a person more likely to become an abuser. A 2005 study of parents of newborns found that couples where one of the spouses had been physically or sexually abused as a child were more than ten times more likely to mistreat their own child.

Finally, child sexual abuse can have long-term effects on both physical and mental health. A 2008 study of the long-term effects of child sexual abuse found that these negative health outcomes lasted well into old age.

Pedophilia is the sexual attraction of an adult to a child. Pedophiles can be any adult with whom a child has contact, including stepparents, teachers, religious leaders, child-care providers, neighbors, babysitters, or doctors. Incest is sexual intercourse between persons too closely related to marry. When it involves a parent or other close relative and a child, incest is a form of pedophilia.

The BJS report on child victims found that 34 percent of the abuse perpetrated on juveniles was by family members. For victims under the age of six, nearly half (49 percent) of all offenders were family member offenders. For juveniles in general, 59 percent of all offenses were committed by non–family members whom the victims knew. Only 7 percent were the acts of strangers.

CHILD PORNOGRAPHY

Child pornography is defined as the visual depiction of an individual under the age of 18 in a sexually explicit manner in any type of publication, picture, or film. The child does not have to be actively engaged in sexual activity; the implication of sexuality is enough for an image to be considered pornography. The U.S. Congress addressed the problem in 1978 by passing the Protection of Children Against Exploitation Act and again in 1986 with the Child Sexual Abuse and Pornography Act. These laws made it a federal crime to engage in child pornography.

Despite these laws, the problem persists. Between March 1998 and September 2003, the Cyber Tipline operated by the National Center for Missing and Exploited Children received 118,987 reports of child pornography and 1,890 reported cases of child prostitution. In 2003, the laws on child pornography were updated once again. The Protect Law made it illegal either to request or offer sexually explicit images of children on the Internet. Interestingly, the law does not require the images to actually exist; simply offering or asking for such images is enough to make a person guilty of a crime. Furthermore, digitally created images or digitally altered images of adults that appear to show children under the age of 18 are also illegal under this law. Although there were objections from several justices, the Supreme Court upheld the law in a 2008 decision.

WHO IS INVOLVED?

Child abusers can be almost anyone, but most are male. According to a 2006 report from the Bureau of Justice Statistics (BJS), nearly all of the offenders in federal child sex exploitation cases were male (97 percent). Female offenders made up only 3 percent of all individuals who were prosecuted for federal sexual exploitation offenses, although they were more likely to be involved in sex trafficking (8.8 percent) than in other crimes such as child pornography (1.3 percent) or sex abuse (3.6 percent). An earlier BJS study found that female offenders were most common in assaults against very young victims, those under the age of six. For these youngest victims, females made up 12 percent of offenders, compared with 6 percent for victims ages six through 12 and 3 percent for victims ages 12 through 17.

Fact Or Fiction?

The people who abuse kids are dirty old men.

The Facts: A considerable percentage of those who abuse children are young themselves. According to a 2006 report, 22 percent of individuals who were federally prosecuted for sexually abusing children were under the age of 21, and another 29 percent were under the age of 30.

According to a detailed BJS study of child victimization, adults were responsible for 67 percent of all assaults on juveniles. However, juveniles were responsible for 40 percent of all assaults on children under the age of six. (Children between the ages of seven and 11 were responsible for 13 percent of these assaults, and teens ranging in age from 12 through 17 were responsible for 27 percent of the assaults.) Researchers found a similar proportion (39 percent) of victims between the ages of six and 11 were also assaulted by other juveniles. In fact, according to a 2006 report from the Bureau of Justice Statistics, 22 percent of federal prosecutions for child sex abuse were of individuals under the age of 21.

See also: Children and Rape; Educating the Community; Help and Support; Internet Predators; Rape Within Abusive Relationships; Statutory Rape

FURTHER READING

Williams, Heidi. *Child Abuse.* San Diego, Calif.: Greenhaven Press, 2009.

Winters, Paul A. *Child Sexual Abuse.* San Diego, Calif.: Greenhaven Press, 1998.

■ STATUTORY RAPE

Sexual intercourse that is defined as **coercive** by law, or statute, because one or both of the participants is below the legal age of consent, usually under 18 years of age. The legal age of **consent** varies not only by state but also by situation. Whether or not a sexual act is considered to be statutory rape may depend not only on the age of the child or teen involved but also on the age of the other sexual partner and the age difference between the perpetrator and the minor. Individuals can be **prosecuted** for statutory rape even if both parties agreed to have sex, because if one or both of them is below the legal age of consent, the law does not consider them to be legally capable of making the decision to have sex.

Statutory rape laws were initially put into place to protect the sexual innocence of young women. Over time, they have become increasingly more **gender neutral** and are now primarily focused on protecting young people from being coerced into having sex. In general, a sexual offense is considered to be statutory rape if it is illegal *only* because of the age of one of the people involved. However, some other types of sexual offenses may be prosecuted as statutory rape, since in such cases, a lack of consent does not need to be proven. As long as it can be proven that the accused has had sex with someone who is under age, that person can be prosecuted for statutory rape.

Fact Or Fiction?

If my 19-year-old boyfriend really believes that I'm 18 instead of 15, then he can't be charged with statutory rape.

The Facts: Just because an adult honestly believes his or her sexual partner to be above the age of consent does not protect him or her from a charge of statutory rape. Even if the young person in question lied about his or her age, in most states it is still possible for an adult who has had sex with a minor to be charged with, and convicted of, statutory rape.

AGE OF CONSENT LAWS

Very few states have laws that simply state, "it is illegal for a person under the age of 12 to have sex." Instead, state laws generally define specific sexual acts that are illegal for individuals of different ages as well as the types of sexual partners who are legally unacceptable. For example, when dealing with **sexual intercourse**, a state may define (1) a *minimum age* below which sexual intercourse is never legal; (2) an *age of consent* where people become legally allowed to consent to sex; (3) how much older a person's sexual partner can legally be, if they are above the minimum age and below the legal age of consent; and (4) the age below which a person cannot be prosecuted for having sex with another minor. The third and fourth concepts are particularly important, because they **decriminalize** sex between two mutually consenting teenagers. Where such distinctions are not in place, it is possible for high-school sweethearts to be jailed for deciding to have sex with each other, even if they are both the same age.

DID YOU KNOW?

State Laws Governing Statutory Rape v. the Legal Age of Consent

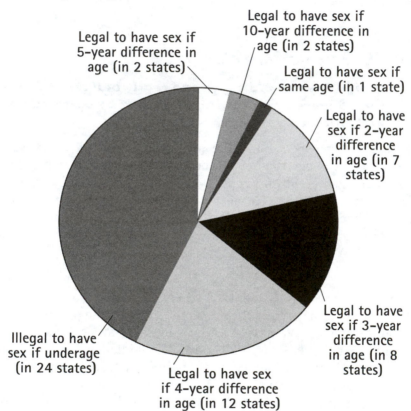

Legal to have sex if 5-year difference in age (in 2 states)

Legal to have sex if 10-year difference in age (in 2 states)

Legal to have sex if same age (in 1 state)

Legal to have sex if 2-year difference in age (in 7 states)

Legal to have sex if 3-year difference in age (in 8 states)

Legal to have sex if 4-year difference in age (in 12 states)

Illegal to have sex if underage (in 24 states)

In 24 states, underage individuals cannot consent to sex, regardless of the difference in age of a partner. However, in 26 states, there are 32 different laws that determine at what age it is legal for a young person to have sex with someone. In Colorado, for example, a girl under 15 can have sex legally with someone who is less than four years older than she, but a 15-17 year old can have sex legally with someone who is up to 10 years older. If the guide is not followed, the act is reported as statutory rape, even if two people are consenting.

Source: *Statutory Rape: A Guide to State Laws and Reporting Requirements*, 2004.

The legal age of consent in the United States ranges from 16 to 18 years of age. As of 2003, 38 states had a minimum age below which no person could ever legally consent to sex. Thirty-five states had no minimum age for prosecution, which means that in those states any individual who has sex with a person below the age of consent can be prosecuted for statutory rape, although in many of those states it is legal to have sex if both partners are within a specified age range of one another or if they are married.

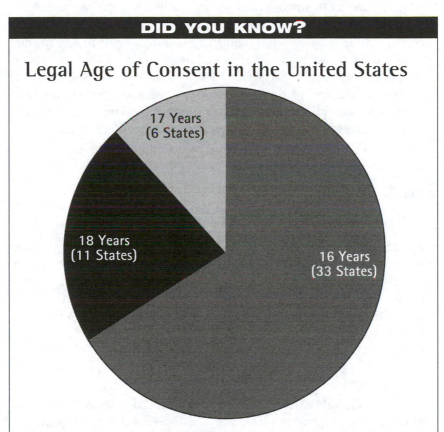

DID YOU KNOW?

Legal Age of Consent in the United States

17 Years
(6 States)

18 Years
(11 States)

16 Years
(33 States)

The legal age of consent varies from state to state. In slightly more than half the states, an individual can legally consent to sex, with no restrictions, starting on his or her 16th birthday. In the rest of the United States, consent is restricted to 17- and 18-year-olds.

Source: The Lewin Group. *Statutory Rape: A Guide to State Laws and Reporting Requirements,* prepared for the Office of the Assistant Secretary for Planning and Evaluation (ASPE), U.S. Department of Health and Human Services (HHS), 2004.

VICTIMS AND OFFENDERS

According to a 2005 report from the Office for Juvenile Justice and Delinquency planning, for every three reported **forcible rapes** against minors there was one reported statutory rape. In the vast majority of cases, the accused was either an acquaintance of the victim, their boyfriend, or their girlfriend.

Most statutory rape victims, 95 percent of them, are female, and 99 percent of the people who offend against female victims are male. Similarly, the vast majority of male statutory rape victims have female partners—94 percent. Men who are involved in a statutory rape incident with a female victim tend to be slightly closer in age to their partners than those who are involved with male victims—six years older instead of nine. In fact, male victims tend to have older partners than female victims, in general. These statistics are not comprehensive because not all states report statutory rape data to the Federal Bureau of Investigation (FBI), but they should provide a reasonable approximation of criminal activity nationwide.

Fact Or Fiction?

Only women are victims of statutory rape.

The Facts: Approximately 5 percent of statutory rape victims are male. The vast majority of the time, more than nine times out of 10, the sexual partners of these young men are female. Interestingly, statutory rape offenders with male victims tend to be older than offenders with female victims. About 70 percent of them are over age 21, and 25 percent are over age 24. In contrast, only 25 percent of offenders with female victims are over 21, and only 25 percent are over 24.

REQUIREMENTS FOR REPORTING

Certain types of professionals are legally required to report any knowledge of child sexual activity so that the possibility of **child abuse** can be investigated. These individuals are known as **mandatory reporters** and reporting requirements vary state by state. In some states, reporting is required only if the person with whom the **minor** is having sex is responsible for their care, such as a parent, teacher, or guardian. In other states, all sexual contact with a minor must be reported to the proper authorities. In general, mandatory reporters are individuals who work with children as part of their jobs, people such as teachers, health-care providers, religious professionals, law enforcement agents, and childcare workers. Reports of statutory rape are usually made to the either local child protection agency or to law enforcement. Those agencies will then investigate the report to see if the minor is in danger or if a crime has been committed.

See also: Abusive Sexual Behavior; Children and Rape; Date Rape; Law and Rape, the; Sexual Violence and Children

TEENS SPEAK

My Boyfriend Was Charged with Statutory Rape

When I was 15, I started dating my best friend's older brother. He was attending a local college and would sometimes come home on the weekends. We had known each other for several years, but we didn't realize that we liked each other until that year.

After we had been together for about six months, we knew we were in love, and we decided to have sex. I had learned all about safe sex in school, and so we decided to use condoms so that I wouldn't have to ask my parents to go to the doctor to get birth control. They liked my boyfriend, but they thought that, at 20, he was a bit too old for me, and I knew that they would not approve of us having sex before we were married.

Normally we were really careful, but one day my mom came into my room and saw an open condom wrapper on the floor by my bed. She got really mad and yelled and screamed at me until I admitted that my boyfriend and I had been having sex for several months. She stormed out of the room and I heard her making a phone call. She had called the police! I heard her telling them that a 20-year-old boy had made her 15-year-old daughter have sex with him and that she wanted him arrested. I started screaming that no one had made me do anything and that I loved him, but she wouldn't let me have the phone.

The next few months were awful. Even though I told the police and the lawyers that I had wanted to have sex with my boyfriend, they still charged him with statutory rape. They said that because I was 15, I didn't know what I wanted and that he should have known better. He did not go to jail, but they said he wasn't allowed to see me again. It didn't matter, since he had dumped me the second he heard my mom had called the police. My best friend hasn't spoken to me since. I still love him, but I wish that all this had never happened.

FURTHER READING
Jellum, Linda D. *Mastering Statutory Interpretation*. Durham, N.C.: Carolina Academic Press, 2008.

■ STIGMA OF RAPE

The burden of shame or disgrace that society may place on someone who has been raped. When people talk about a crime being "stigmatized," they mean that society may look down on, or otherwise judge, the victim for having been victimized. The continued judgment of, or disdain for, victims of rape is a form of social stigmatization. Unfortunately, it is not uncommon for victims of rape or sexual assault to suffer not just from the attack but also from their treatment by their friends and relatives afterwards. They may be seen as somehow being contaminated by the assault and treated differently in a way that only increases the trauma resulting from the attack. This is one of the reasons why many rape victims do not report their attack. They are ashamed of what happened to them, even though it is in no way their fault.

PSYCHOLOGICAL IMPACT

If you are sexually assaulted, you may experience psychological effects as a direct result of the trauma associated with that attack. You may also experience psychological effects related to the potential stigma of the attack, or the shame you might feel. The loss of, or feeling that you have lost, the respect of those you care about can be very difficult. Some teenagers also feel embarrassment in the eyes of their peers. The myths surrounding rape can cause you to worry that your friends or teachers will think you somehow asked to be raped or that things did not happen the way you said they did. If you were assaulted by someone else in your school or social circle, you must also contend with his or her friends and their feelings about someone they know getting him or her in trouble.

As a rape victim, you may begin to question your judgment about everyone. This may be particularly true if you were raped by someone you know. You may try to avoid situations that remind you of the attack, even to the point of not being able to live your life fully. Your friends and family may be of little help. They may feel embarrassed, helpless, or angry. They may avoid you because they do not want to be reminded of their own vulnerability. You may well feel lonely and alone, and this can lead to depression and feelings of low self-esteem.

Stigma and fears related to disclosure may contribute to a reluctance to report a sexual assault or to receive help for it afterward. Those who keep silent about their sexual assault often do not heal as fast or as thoroughly as those who are able to talk about it with supportive people, namely professionals, friends, and family. Reporting the crime can give you a sense of control and empowerment. Receiving help can give you a release of pent-up despair and can teach you skills to manage your emotions. If you allow the fear of stigma to keep you from talking about your ordeal, you are more likely to continue to experience depression, anxiety, flashbacks, or memory problems.

However, while the emotional scars of a sexual assault are very real, it does not follow that every time you have physical symptoms it is related to that trauma. Unfortunately, medical personnel sometimes assume that any physical problems manifested by a sexual assault victim are related to their psychological state. If your doctor knows your history, he or she may be inclined to dismiss any illness on the basis that it must be **psychosomatic** (caused by your mind) or "all in your head." If a person truly thinks something is wrong, he or she should not accept the diagnosis of stress, and make sure to get a second opinion.

TEENS SPEAK

I Would Do It Again

When I was 12 years old my mother's boyfriend started molesting me. I told my mom but she didn't do a thing about it. I wanted to tell someone else, but I just couldn't bring myself to do it. I thought I would be blamed and ignored, even though I knew it was real.

Apparently my little sister said something to her teacher after a presentation in her class. I'm not sure exactly what she said, but it got her teacher's attention. She phoned authorities right away, and they came right to my classroom and pulled me out, during class. I was told by a police officer and a social worker they needed to discuss a very important matter. It was kind of embarrassing because I thought I had done something very, very wrong. My whole class was watching while I tried to tell myself that it couldn't be about that. I was sure nobody knew because I hadn't told anybody.

I was taken to the nurse's room, which was the only place we could have this kind of interview, and I remained there for seven hours as I gave my statement, through anger and tears. Not long after that I found myself in court. I was only 12 and testifying against an "adult" who was also my mother's boyfriend.

He was found guilty on five counts of sexual assault and sentenced to five years in prison. In the end, though, he only spent a couple years there after he received counseling and was released on good behavior. I would still do it again, though. It's only by telling our stories that others will realize how much damage these people do to our lives. I am convinced that our voices will change the course of justice—as long as we keep telling our stories.

LEGAL IMPACT

Many victims fear that they will be shamed and humiliated if they go through the legal process after reporting their rape. A rape victim must submit to an intrusive and sometimes painful medical exam after the assault in order to collect physical evidence. She or he must retell the story, sometimes many times, to police and prosecutors. Depending on the specifics of the case and their own prejudices, law enforcement personnel may not believe all or part of a victim's story or may act as though they do not believe it in order to make sure he or she does not change the story. They may be particularly tough if the victim has no bruises or other evidence of physical resistance. If the victim knows the assailant or has waited a long time to report the rape, they may also give him or her a harder time. Because of these facts and the fears of victims, with more than half of rapes going unreported. Rape victims who do come forward are brave to do so, and they help ensure, at their own risk, that the rapist will not be able to attack anyone else. Remember the rapist has committed a crime; he is to blame, not the victim, regardless of the circumstances surrounding the assault.

Fact Or Fiction?

Unless a weapon is used it isn't really rape.

The Facts: Anytime someone forces intercourse, it is rape. The force may include the use of weapons, threats or intimidation, drugs, alcohol, or a victim's own diminished mental capacity.

COURT APPEARANCES

Victims of rape have to appear in court to testify against their assailant. Many rape victims find this extremely difficult. They not only have to tell their story in front of a judge, the defendant, his lawyer, the jury, and any observers but also need to be prepared to defend themselves against the questions of the defendant's lawyer. This lawyer will attempt to pick apart the victim's story and, to the extent allowed by law, will try to suggest that he or she is not a **credible** witness or that he or she is not telling the truth. This can be humiliating and degrading, as the lawyers may bring things up that most people would prefer not to reveal in public. Victims will have to face their assailant as well, as he has a legal right to be present while they are testifying. This can be especially difficult if the two knew each other before the attack, even though the assailant will not be permitted to speak to his accuser.

It is important to find out beforehand what resources are available to those who testify in a court of law. Some sexual assault crisis centers will retain an attorney to help survivors navigate the legal system or will suggest someone who can help them understand the workings of the court and tell them what to expect. Most courts have a victim's advocate who can help survivors through the process, including providing them with compensation information and court support. Survivors can also ask to be notified of other court appearances where their assailant must appear, but they do not have to go to these unless they want.

Q & A

Question: Why do some people believe that a person "asked to be raped"?

Answer: It can sometimes be difficult for some people to determine what constitutes consent in the context of sexual behavior. Some believe that when a woman dresses in revealing clothing, dances in a way that imitates sexual closeness, or flirts, she is encouraging sexual advances. Such behavior usually only means that a woman wants to be noticed, however, and not that she necessarily wants to have sex. None of these behaviors gives anyone the right to assume that a woman wants sex or that it is acceptable to force themselves on her.

Those who do not want to testify can ask the prosecutor to pursue a **plea bargain**, where the attacker will be offered an opportunity to plead guilty to a lesser charge without a trial. Some victims find this easier than waiting a year or more for a trial, testifying, and then taking the risk that the attacker will be **acquitted**, or found not guilty. Others prefer to do whatever it takes for the rapist to end up in jail for the longest possible time period. To the extent they can, victims should try to do what feels most comfortable for them. They should not let themselves be pressured by the expectations of their family, law enforcement, friends, or society at large. The trial, however, is the state's case, not theirs. Therefore, the ultimate decision whether or not to pursue a plea bargain with the defendant is up to the prosecuting attorney. Depending on the circumstances of the case, it is possible that the prosecutor will enter into a plea agreement even against a victim's wishes. However, it is important

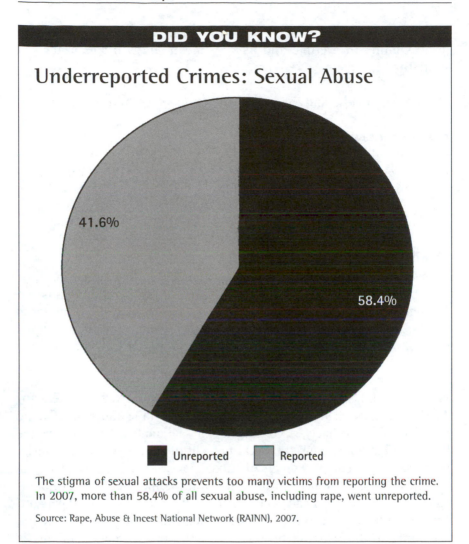

DID YOU KNOW?

Underreported Crimes: Sexual Abuse

41.6%

58.4%

■ Unreported   ■ Reported

The stigma of sexual attacks prevents too many victims from reporting the crime. In 2007, more than 58.4% of all sexual abuse, including rape, went unreported.

Source: Rape, Abuse & Incest National Network (RAINN), 2007.

policies of recent years, including longer sentences, three-strikes laws, and mandatory minimums mean fewer criminals overall are on the streets. Because rapists commit many kinds of crimes, and because all kinds of criminals commit rape, locking up an armed robber or drug dealer will often prevent future sexual assaults according to Scott Berkowitz, president and founder of the Rape, Abuse and Incest National Network (RAINN), America's largest anti–sexual assault organization.

to know that plea agreement still means the assailant has admitte
he was guilty of a crime and usually means he will spend at leas
some time in prison.

See also: Rape Kits and Evidence Collection; Rape and Society

FURTHER READING

Feuereisen, Patti. *Invisible Girls: The Truth About Sexual Abuse—A Book for Teen Girls, Young Women, and Everyone Who Cares About Them.* New York: Seal Press, 2005.

■ VICTIMS OF RAPE: FEMALE

Women who are forced or coerced into engaging in vaginal, oral, or anal intercourse are victims of rape. Nine out of 10 rape victims are women. Almost all are raped by a man. In most cases, the offender is known to the victim. Rape usually involves penetration of a victim's vagina, mouth, or anus with a penis, other body part, or object.

REPORTING

Women of all backgrounds and ethnicities are raped. Native American/ Alaska Native women are most likely to report a rape and Asian/Pacific Islanders the least likely, according to the National Institute of Justice in 1998. This study showed that 34 percent of Native American/Alaska Natives, 24 percent of women of mixed race, 19 percent of African-American women, 18 percent of white women, and 8 percent of Asian/ Pacific Islander women had been raped. Almost all rapes, 80–90 percent, are committed by someone of the same racial background as the victim, according to the Department of Justice. The one exception to this is Native American victims of rape, who reported in 1997 that the offender was either white or African American in 90 percent of the attacks.

CHANGING ATTITUDES

The number of incidents of rape, attempted rape, and sexual assault declined by more than 17 percent between 1996 and 2006. This decline was even more marked in the first few years of this century. Experts believe two trends are largely responsible for the tremendous decline in sexual violence over the last decade. First, tough-on-crime

DID YOU KNOW?

Age of First Sexual Assault

Age Range (Years)	Percent of Victims (Female)	Percent of Victims (Male)
<12	25	41
12–17	35	28
18–24	28	19
>25	11	12

In short, 25 percent of women and 41 percent of men who are sexually assaulted experience their first assault before the age of 12; 35 percent of women and 28 percent of men are first assaulted between the ages of 12 and 17.

Source: Basile, et. al., *Violence and Victims 22* (4); 437–448, 2007.

The second trend is generational. Rape victims are overwhelmingly young, and this generation has grown up being taught that "No Means No." Young women today are both more careful about entering into potentially dangerous situations and more willing to forcefully express their own desires. Increased media attention and a greater societal openness about sexual matters are also likely factors in an increased willingness to report sexual assaults to police.

More and more survivors of sexual assault are speaking out publicly, helping to lessen the stigma long associated with rape victims. A higher proportion of rapes are reported than in the past, as women learn to speak out about what has happened to them. Advocates, prosecutors, and survivors are also working together in states across the country to change laws and statutes to make rape prosecutions more effective.

See also: Help and Support; Rape Statistics; Stigma of Rape; Victims of Rape: Male

FURTHER READING

Buchwald, Emilie, Pamela R. Fletcher, and Martha Roth. *Transforming a Rape Culture*. Minneapolis: Milkweed Editions, 2005.

■ VICTIMS OF RAPE: MALE

Men who are forced or coerced into engaging in oral or anal intercourse or any other form of nonconsensual sexual activity are victims of male rape. According to the National Center for Victims of Crime, boys in their early and mid-teens are more likely to be victimized than older males, with victims averaging 17 years of age.

Male rape usually involves penetration of a victim's mouth or anus with a penis, other body part, or object. The assault may also take the form of gang rape, which is more common in cases involving male victims than those involving females. Perpetrators who attack men are likely to demand multiple sex acts and are more likely to display weapons as a threat and to use them than those who assault women. Therefore, male victims face a greater risk of being injured physically, and their injuries are often more serious than those suffered by female rape victims.

Although forcing sex on a man is a crime in every state, in many jurisdictions, it is not considered rape but is placed under the broader term *sexual assault.* Many rape laws are gender-specific, defining rape as a crime against women only. However, this is simply an issue of legal definitions. Men can still be victims of rape.

STATISTICS

According to the 2005 National Crime Victimization Survey, Americans reported 176,540 incidences of rape and other sexual assaults involving female victims and 15,130 incidences involving male victims, or 191,670 total cases, down from previous years. The survey estimates that in about 30 percent of these cases, the offender was an intimate partner and in 44 percent, an acquaintance or friend.

According to a 2007 report, 13.8 million Americans—11 percent of women and 3 percent of men—have experienced forced sex at least once in their lifetime. A 2000 report on sex offenses and offenders issued by the U.S. Bureau of Justice Statistics points out that males face the greatest risk of sexual assault at age four. By the time a male becomes a teenager, his risk of sexual assault is only one-10th that of adolescent females, who face the highest risk of assault.

A common misconception among the public is that male rape is a homosexual crime. While rape is often used as a hate crime against gay men, neither the victims nor the perpetrators are necessarily gay. In a 1980 study of victims and offenders published in the *American Journal of Psychiatry*, half of the offenders and victims described their consenting sexual encounters as heterosexual. An additional 38 percent had consenting sexual encounters with both men and women. About half of the offenders did not consider the gender of the victim important. Instead, they appeared to be relatively indiscriminate when it came to their choice of a victim. Their victims included males and females as well as adults and children. Perhaps not surprisingly, attackers who prefer younger victims are just as likely to prefer to attack either gender, boys or girls. A 2008 study in the journal *Sexual Abuse* found that individuals who had abused a victim under the age of six were three times more likely to abuse victims of both genders than those individuals who only assaulted older children.

The 1980 study was part of the background research for a second study, in 2001, on assaults of adult males published in the *Journal of Interpersonal Violence*. Researchers found that male victims of sexual assault tended to be young, single men who were particularly vulnerable. Some were homeless; others had physical, psychiatric, or mental disabilities.

REPORTING

Generally, embarrassment, shame, and fear tend to make victims unwilling to come forward and report sex crimes. This is certainly true of female victims and may be even more pronounced among male victims. In the 1980 victim/offender study in the *American Journal of Psychiatry*, a major reason male rape appeared to be underreported was the stigma associated with it.

A 2006 report on male disclosure of sexual abuse and rape also discusses other reasons that men may underreport sexual assaults, including the belief that they are not supposed to be strongly affected by rape and the fear that an involuntary sexual response to the experience may lead them to be thought of as homosexual.

Like women who have been raped, male victims tend to blame themselves. The National Center for Victims of Crime notes that a major concern of male rape victims is society's belief that men should be able to protect themselves and, therefore, it is somehow their fault that they were raped.

Numerous studies support this idea that male victims of rape, particularly gay male victims of rape, are more likely to be blamed for their rape. Interestingly, one 2008 paper in the *Journal of Homosexuality* found that individuals were more likely to blame a heterosexual male rape victim for the attack if he did fight back and a homosexual male rape victim if he did not. For men, a rape may challenge the view that they can take care of themselves physically and mentally and raise questions about their masculinity. This leads to another reason that many men are afraid to report being the victim of a sexual assault, they are concerned that they will be labeled as homosexual.

CHANGING ATTITUDES

Attitudes toward sexual assault change with the times. Perhaps the easiest way to gauge the change in attitude on male rape is to consider the titles of two academic articles on the subject, separated by almost 50 years. According to 2001 training material from the National Center for Women and Policing, sexual assault treatment centers report that males make up approximately 6–10 percent of their clients. A 2008 study in the *Journal of Emergency Medicine* reported that approximately 8 percent of all sexual assault cases in one large urban emergency department were males.

In 2007, a multinational study of sexual coercion among university students found that 3 percent of male participants reported being forced to have sex and 22 percent reported verbal coercion about sexual issues. Men were most often coerced into having sex without a condom (14 percent) but also threatened or coerced into vaginal sex, oral sex, and anal sex. Coercion was more common in longer relationships and in relationships where sex was already occurring. Men were also at greater risk of experiencing sexual coercion if they had been abused as children or saw themselves as being low on the social desirability scale.

While public understanding of the male rape problem has slowly grown, neither victims nor society as a whole finds it easy to deal with the situation. One advance is that several state governments have revised their rape laws to make them gender-neutral. Hopefully, expanding knowledge of the problem will enable better reporting and more opportunities for victims to seek treatment without unnecessary shame.

See also: Children and Rape; Help and Support; Rape and Society; Rape Statistics; Stigma of Rape; Victims of Rape: Female

FURTHER READING
Abdullah-Khan, Noreen *Male Rape: The Emergence of a Social and Legal Issue.* New York: Palgrave Macmillan, 2008.

Atkinson, Matt. *Resurrection After Rape: A Guide to Transforming from Victim to Survivor.* Oklahoma City, Oklahoma: R.A.R. Publishing, 2008.
La Valle, John. *Everything You Need to Know When You Are the Male Survivor of Rape or Sexual Assault.* New York: Rosen Publishing Group, 1996.

HOTLINES
AND HELP SITES

Child Welfare League of America
URL: http://www.cwla.org
Phone: (703) 412-2400
Fax: (703) 412-2401
Address: 2345 Crystal Drive, Suite 250, Arlington, VA 22202
Mission: To promote the well-being of children, youths, and their families and to protect every child from harm

Girls Incorporated
URL: http://girlsinc.org
Phone: (800) 374-4475; (212) 509-2000
Fax: (212) 509-8708
Address: 120 Wall Street, Third Floor, New York, NY 10005
E-mail: Communications@girlsinc.org
Mission: To help every girl become strong, smart, and bold through advocacy, research, and education

National Center for HIV, STD and TB Prevention
Affiliation: Centers for Disease Control and Prevention
URL: http://www.cdc.gov/nchstp/od/nchstp.html
Phone: (800) CDC-INFO (800-232-4636, for information on STD clinics and testing); (800) 342-AIDS
Address: 1600 Clifton Road, Atlanta, GA 90333
E-mail: cdcinfo@cdc.gov
Mission: To provide health information on sexually transmitted diseases and other diseases

National Center for Missing and Exploited Children
URL: http://www.missingkids.com
Phone: (800) THE-LOST (843-5678)
Fax: (703) 274-2200
Address: Charles B. Wang International Children's Building, 699 Prince Street, Alexandria, VA 22314-3175
Mission: To provide services nationwide for families and professionals in the prevention of abducted, endangered, and sexually exploited children. Also to provide a way to securely report child sexual abuse online using the cybertipline.

National Child Abuse Hotline
URL: http://www.childhelp.org
Phone: (800) 4-A-CHILD (422-4453)
Mission: To meet the physical, emotional, educational, and spiritual needs of abused and neglected children

The National Children's Advocacy Center (NCAC)
URL: http://www.nationalcac.org
Phone: (256) 533-5437
Fax: (256) 534-6883
Address: 210 Pratt Avenue, Huntsville, AL 35801
Mission: To provide prevention, intervention, and treatment services to physically and sexually abused children and their families by using a child-focused team approach

National Domestic Violence Hotline
Project of the Texas Council on Family Violence
URL: http://www.ndvh.org
Phone: (800) 799-SAFE (7233); (800) 787-3224 (TTY)
Mission: To provide victims of domestic abuse with 24-hour, 365-day access; more than 4,000 shelters and service providers are located across the country including Alaska, Hawaii, and the U.S. Virgin Islands

National Women's Health Information Center
U.S. Department of Health and Human Services
URL: http://www.4woman.gov
Phone: (800) 994-WOMAN (9662); (888) 220-5446 (TDD)
Mission: To provide free, reliable health information for women everywhere, including a database of resources and topics such as heart disease, disabilities, and pregnancy

Prevent Child Abuse America
URL: http://www.preventchildabuse.com
Phone: (800) CHILDREN (800-244-5373); (312) 663-3520
Fax: (312) 939-8962
Address: 500 North Michigan Avenue, Suite 200, Chicago, IL 60611-3703
Email: mailbox@preventchildabuse.org
Mission: To build awareness, provide education, and inspire hope to everyone involved in the effort to prevent the abuse and neglect of children

Rape, Abuse & Incest National Network (RAINN)
URL: http://www.rainn.org
Address: 200 L Street, Washington, DC 20036
Phone: (800) 656-HOPE (4673)
Fax: (202) 544-3556
E-mail: info@rainn.org
Program: Operates a 24-hour confidential national hotline for survivors of sexual assault

The Safer Society Foundation
URL: http://www.safersociety.org
Phone: (802) 247-3132
Fax: (802) 247-4233
Address: P.O. Box 340, Brandon, VT 05733-0340
Mission: To advocate the prevention and treatment of sexual abuse. The foundation focuses primarily on the treatment of offenders and offers publications on sexual abuse and therapist referrals for offenders.

Safe School Helpline
URL: http://www.schoolhelpline.com
Phone: (800) 325-4381
Fax: (614) 760-2828
Mission: To provide a 24-hour service that empowers students, parents, and community members to report unsafe, at-risk situations without identifying themselves

The Sexuality Information and Education Council of the United States
URL: http://www.siecus.org
Phone: (212) 819-9770 (NY office); (202) 265-2405 (Washington, D.C., office)

Fax: (212) 819-9776; (202) 462-2340

Address: 90 John St., Suite 704, New York, NY 10038; 1706 R Street, Washington, DC 20009

Mission: To affirm that sexuality is a natural and healthy part of living; to develop, collect, and disseminate information; to promote comprehensive education about sexuality; and to advocate the right of individuals to make responsible sexual choices

Survivors of Incest Anonymous

URL: http://www.siawso.org

Phone: (410) 893-3322

Address: P.O. Box 190, Benson, MD 21018

E-mail: siawso.info@gmail.com

Mission: To provide information on incest and child sexual abuse as well as referrals to local support groups

Women's Health America

URL: http://www.womenshealth.com

Phone: (800) 558-7046

Fax: (888) 898-7412

Address: 1289 Demming Way, Madison, WI 53717

Mission: To provide resources necessary for women to make sound, well-informed health-care choices

Youth Risk Behavior Surveillance System

URL: http://www.cdc.gov/yrbs

Affiliation: Centers for Disease Control's National Center for Chronic Disease Prevention and Health Promotion

Mission: To monitor priority health risk behaviors that contribute markedly to the leading causes of death, disability, and social problems among youths and adults in the United States

GLOSSARY

acquaintance rape sexual assaults committed by someone known to the victim, such as a date, teacher, employer, or family member. Date rape is a specific type of acquaintance rape.

age of consent the minimum age for consensual sexual relations; depending on the state, the age of consent varies from 14 to 18 years of age

antiretroviral drugs drugs used to treat retroviruses, particularly HIV

anus opening at the lower end of the alimentary canal

assailant a person who attacks another

assault intentionally inflicting harm on another

celibacy the state of abstaining from sexual intercourse

chain of evidence the record of how a piece of evidence, or proof, was handled from the moment it was collected until it arrives in a court of law

child abuse the physical, sexual, or emotional mistreatment of a child

child molester a person who sexually abuses a child

clitoral hood   the flap of skin covering the clitoris

clitoris   the erectile organ of the female genital tract

coercive   forced

cohabitate   to live with someone without being legally married

colposcopy   a technique that is used to obtain a magnified view of the genitalia

compliance   willingness to submit to the will of another; may mean saying "yes" when you mean no

conception   the fertilization of an egg by a sperm; the onset of pregnancy

connotation   a suggestion different from a term's explicit meaning

consensual   something that has been consented or agreed to

consent   permission

conviction   the state of being found guilty for one's actions in a court of law

decriminalization   the process of removing, or reducing, legal consequences for a criminal action

deviations   sexual behaviors that result, in part, from an inability to establish normal sexual relationships

DNA   the genetic information essential to living cells that controls inherited characteristics

domestic violence   physical or sexual violence or psychological abuse committed by family members or intimate partners

emergency contraception   drugs used to prevent a woman from becoming pregnant after she has had unprotected sex

exhibitionism   exposure of the genitals to non-consenting individuals

felony   a serious crime punishable by death or imprisonment for more than one year. Arson, burglary, murder, and rape are all felonies.

fetus   the developing product of conception, from about eight weeks until birth

fondling   to caress or handle in a manner showing desire

forcible rape   sexual activity, or attempts at such activity, which take place against a person's will

gender neutral   when the state of being male or female is irrelevant

gender-based violence   attacks on people because of their gender, for example, violence against women

genetic   hereditary

genitalia   reproductive organs

GHB   gamma hydroxybutyrate; a colorless and odorless depressant that acts on the central nervous system; used in date rapes

heredity   the transmission of characteristics from parents to offspring

heterosexual   one who directs sexual desires toward the opposite sex

homosexual   one who directs sexual desires toward the same sex

incest   sexual intercourse between persons forbidden by law to marry because they are closely related

intimacy   close or warm friendship

intimidation   threatening someone to gain control over that person

labia majora   the outer folds of skin that are part of the external female genital tract

labia minora   the inner folds of skin which are part of the external female genital tract

leering   looking at a person in a sexual way

lust   an intense sexual desire or need

mandatory reporter   an individual who is required by law to report any suspicion of a crime

marital rape   when a wife is raped by her husband

metabolize   to process by the body

minor   a person who is legally considered to be a child

molest   to make improper sexual advances; to force sexual contact

molester   one who touches another in an improper sexual manner with intent to harm; see also **child molester**

nonconsensual   without consent

objectify   to talk about a person in a manner that suggests they do not have feelings or value

parole board   law enforcement personnel and others who can consider the release of a prisoner before his or her sentence has expired, based on good behavior

pedophile   a person who is sexually attracted to children

perpetrator   one who commits a crime against another

plea bargain   agreement in which a perpetrator is offered the opportunity to plead guilty to a lesser charge without a trial

pornography   the production of writings, pictures, or films of people performing sex acts; media with no artistic value other than to stimulate sexual desire

post-traumatic stress disorder (PTSD) syndrome characterized by reliving a trauma in memories and dreams, avoiding anything reminiscent of the event, memory loss, emotional numbing, sleep disturbance, anxiety, severe depression, and alcohol and substance abuse

promiscuity having sexual relationships with many different individuals without a significant attachment toward anyone

prophylactic preventing or guarding against disease; a condom

prophylaxis taking medication to reduce the likelihood of acquiring a disease

prosecute to pursue justice in a court of law

psychosomatic describes a physical condition that is influenced by psychological or emotional factors

rape trauma syndrome illness whereby an abused partner suffers from shock, memory loss, nightmares, reliving the incident(s) over and over, helplessness, anxiety, and depression

rapist one who is guilty of forcing sexual intercourse through the use of coercion

Rohypnol a powerful sedative sometimes known as roofies, rophies, roach, and rope; known as a date rape drug

sex offender one who has been convicted of a sex crime

sexual assault any unwanted sexual contact or attention without consent

sexual battery rape; oral, anal, or vaginal penetration by another without consent

sexual intercourse a form of sexual activity that involves penetration by the penis

sociopath   one who has no regard for the safety, health, or well-being of others and takes advantage of them with no remorse

sodomy   anal intercourse

statutory rape   sex with someone who is under the age of consent, ranging from 14 to 18 years of age, depending on the state

stranger rape   sexual assault by someone the victim does not know

suggestive behavior   acts that stimulate sexual thoughts

token resistance   saying "no" when "yes" is what is actually meant

trauma   emotional and physical shock

virility   the quality or state of vigorous manhood; sexually potent

voyeurism   a practice in which a person receives sexual gratification by watching others nude or having sexual intercourse without their knowledge

vulva   the external genital organs of a female

INDEX

Entries and page numbers in **boldface** indicate major treatment of a topic.

A

abortion 96–98. *See also* emergency contraception
abusive relationships, rape within **123–128**
  child abuse 126–127
  date rape 127–128
  partner abuse 123–126
abusive sexual behavior **15–19**
  heredity and environmental influences 18–19
  psychological impairments 17–18
  social influences 15–16
  social skills, deficient 16–17
acquaintance rape. *See* date rape
Adam Walsh Child Protection and Safety Act 103
age of consent. *See* statutory rape
Aggressive Behavior 77
Alan Guttmacher Institute 23
alcohol and rape. *See* drugs, alcohol, and rape
Allison, Julie 77
alprazolam (Xanax) 31
American Academy of Child and Adolescent Psychiatry 127
American Association of University Women 146–149
American Journal of Health Studies 82
American Journal of Preventive Medicine 27
American Journal of Psychiatry 168–169
Amnesty International 109, 110
Annals of Sex Research 77
Annals of the New York Academy of Science 77
Ativan (lorazepam) 31

B

Benadryl 31
Benedict XVI (pope) 97
Berkowitz, Scott 166
Bohmer, Carol 55
Bryant, Kobe 82
Bureau of Justice Statistics
  children and sexual violence 135, 151
  date rape 26
  incarceration of rapists 8
  intimate partner violence 125
  male victims 168
  prisons, rapes in 135
  rape rates 85
  school safety 130

C

Catholic Church 96–98
CDC. *See* Centers for Disease Control
and Prevention (CDC) 44, 78, 117
CEMC. *See* National Center for
Missing and Exploited Children
Census Bureau, U.S. 64
Centers for Disease Control and
Prevention (CDC) 44, 78, 117
Chamberlain, Wilt 82
Child Abuse & Neglect 17
children and rape 19–25
and abusive relationships
126–127
encouraging nonviolent behavior
20–21
prevention strategies 22–23
sexual assault of children, defined
144
support for children and parents
60–61
teens and rape 23–24
children and sexual violence
151–154
Child Sexual Abuse and Pornography
Act 152
Child Welfare League of America
173
Church of Jesus Christ of Latter-day
Saints 48
circumcision, female 51–52
Clinical Psychology Review 17
clonazepam (Klonopin) 31
club drugs 31, 39–40, 62, 141–142
Coalition for Juvenile Justice 136
college rapes
and date rape 26, 140
fraternities and binge drinking
80–82
and gang rape 55–57
statistics 117
College Student Journal 82
Commonwealth Fund 53

Crandall, C. 115
CyberTipline 70, 153

D

date rape 25–36
and abusive relationships 127–128
v. consensual sex 24
contributing factors 28–32
defined 5, 140
drugs used in 31, 39–40, 62
help for victims 33–36
preventing 32–33
statistics 26–27, 80
date rape drugs 31, 39–40, 62
Debbie Smith Act 115
Declaration on the Elimination of
Violence Against Women (UN) 52
Defense, U.S. Department of
alcohol and rape 35
child abuse 126
children and sexual violence
151–152
college rapes 26
date rape 26, 35
gang rape 53
gender of victims and perpetrators
60
male role in rape 75
media and rape 107
prisoners' history of abuse 137
rape rates 6, 85
school safety 130
sexual assault nurse examiners
(SANE) 115
DNA 42. *See also* evidence
collection and rape kits
domestic violence. *See* intimate
partner violence
dress restrictions 29, 47–49
drugs, alcohol, and rape 36–41
alcohol and sexual violence
37–39, 119
binge drinking and rape 81

and date rape 30–32, 80
drug-facilitated rape 141–142
drugs and sexual violence 39–41, 119
statistics 35

E

ecstasy 39
educating the community **41–46**
friends, educating 89–90
other groups 45–46
police awareness 42–43
and prevention 84
safety concerns 133–134
school programs 43–45
Education, U.S. Department of 130, 147, 149
elder abuse 138–139
emergency contraception 96, 114. *See also* abortion
Ensler, Eve 51
ethnicity and rape 165
evidence collection and rape kits **111–116**
collecting evidence 42, 111–113
sexual assault nurse examiners 114
unprocessed kits 114–115
exhibitionism 64, 144

F

Faces of Violence in Schools (Sandhu) 146
fact or fiction
alcohol and rape 39
child abusers 153
children and sexual abuse 23
evidence collection 113–114
fighting an attacker 93
gang rape 54
gender and sexual abuse 22–23
Internet safety 69

marital rape 125
media and rape 106
prevention 88
prisons, rape in 136
rapists 15, 120
reporting rape 43, 59, 131
sex drive and rape 78
sexual harassment 145, 148
statutory rape 155, 158
victims of rape 30, 74–75
war, rape in 108–109
weapons in rape 163
Federal Bureau of Investigation (FBI)
date rape 25
intimate partner violence 125
men as victims 123
rapists 18
statutory rape 158
Federal Rules of Evidence 73
Female Power and Male Dominance (Sanday) 99
female rights **46–53**
dress restrictions 47–49
genital mutilation 51–52
honor killings 52–53
sex segregation in Israel 49–50
sexual freedom 47
Take Back the Night rallies 50
females. *See* female rights; victims of rape, female
Finkelhor, D. 65
flunitrazepam (Rohypnol) 31, 40, 62, 142
fraternities. *See* college rapes
Fromme and Wendel 38

G

gamma hydroxybutyrate (GHB) 31, 39, 40, 62, 141–142
gang rape **53–58**
and athletes 82
on college campuses 55
preventing 56–57

protection from 57
rapists, characteristics of 54
Gender and Society 80–81
gender roles 3–4, 9–10, 15–16,
78–79, 100–101
genetics 18–19
Geneva Convention 111
genital mutilation 51–52
GHB (gamma hydroxybutyrate) 31,
39, 40, 62, 141–142
Girls Incorporated 173
Glaser, William 16
Groth, A. Nicholas 77

H

Harrington and Leitenberg 37
Harvard School of Public Health 81
Harvey, Mary R. 26
Health and Human Services, U.S.
Department of 20, 22–23, 117–118,
151, 157
Helitzer, D. 115
help and support **58–63**
for children 60–61
date rape victims 33–36
law enforcement 59–60
for parents 61
responding to rape 61–63
support groups 58
heredity 18–19
honor killings 52–53
Hostile Hallways 146–147

I

*Impact Evaluation of a Sexual
Assault Nurse Examiner (SANE)*
(Crandall & Helitzer) 115
incest 141, 152
I Never Called It Rape (Warshaw) 54
institutions, sexual abuse in
134–139
juvenile detention facilities
136–138

mental institutions 134–135
nursing homes 138–139
prisons 135–136
International Women's Day 104
The Internet and the Family study
68
Internet predators **64–71**. *See also*
rapists
finding victims 66–68
meeting Internet acquaintances
70–71
safety on the Internet 68–70
sexual abuse on the Internet
64–66
intimate partner violence 99,
123–126, 129–130. *See also* marital
rape
I-Safe 70
Islam 48, 98, 109–110
Israel, sex segregation in 49–50

J

Johnson, Carl 82
Johnson, Magic (Earvin) 82
Journal of Adolescence 21
*Journal of Consulting Clinical
Psychology* 83
Journal of Developmental Psychology
21
Journal of Emergency Medicine
170
Journal of Homosexuality 169–170
Journal of Interpersonal Violence
121, 169
*Journal of Pediatric and Adolescent
Gynecology* 27
Journal of School Health 81
Journal of Sex Research 17
Journal of Social Issues 76
Journal of Sport and Social Issues
82
Journal of Studies on Alcohol 37
Judaism 48–49, 98

Justice, U.S. Department of 82
  alcohol and rape 35
  child abuse 126
  children and sexual violence
    151–152
  college rapes 26
  date rape 26, 35
  gang rape 53
  gender of victims and perpetrators
    60
  male role in rape 75
  media and rape 107
  prisoners' history of abuse 137
  rape rates 6, 85
  school safety 130
  sexual assault nurse examiners
    (SANE) 115

Justice for All 115
juvenile detention facilities
  136–137
Juvenile Forensic Evaluation
  Resource Center 138

K
Ketalan (ketamine) 31, 39–40
ketamine (Ketalan) 31, 39–40
Klonopin (clonazepam) 31
Koss, Mary P. 26, 28, 30

L
law and rape 71–75
  child pornography 152–153
  evidence collection 115
  legal impact of rape 162–163
  Megan's Laws 103
  newspaper reports of rape 105
  police awareness 42–43
  prisons, rape in 136
  shield laws 73–74, 106
  statutory rape 155–158
  and support for victims 59–60
  war, rape in 111

Lenssen, Phillip 6
Lewin Group 157
lorazepam (Ativan) 31

M
male role in rape **75–83**. *See also*
  rapists; victims of rape, male
  reasons for rape 75–77
  situational factors 80–83
  socialization 77–80
mandatory reporters 158–159
marital rape 5–6, 101–102, 125, 128,
  140–141. *See also* intimate partner
  violence
Martin, Patricia Yancey 57
Mayo Clinic 31
media and rape **105–108**
Megan's Laws 103
mental institutions 134–135
*Men Who Rape: The Psychology of
  the Offender* (Groth) 77
military, rapes in 82
Minnesota Student Survey 27
Mitchell, K. 65
Model Mugging 88
Mormonism 48
myths of rape 8–10

N
Nadeau, Larry 88
National Center for Education
  Statistics 130, 131
National Center for HIV, STD, and TB
  Prevention 173
National Center for Missing and
  Exploited Children (CEMC)
  contact information 174
  CyberTipline 70, 153
  Internet predators 64–65
  Online Victimization Survey 66
  prevention strategies 22
  reporting abuse 61

National Center for Victims of Crime
  child sexual abuse 151
  male victims 168, 169
  reporting rape 36
  shield laws 73–74
National Center for Women and Girls
  in Education 150
National Center for Women and
  Policing 170
National Child Abuse Hotline
  174
National Children's Advocacy Center
  (NCAC) 174
National College Women Sexual
  Victimization Study 117
National Crime Victimization Survey
  male victims 168
  rape rates 7, 85, 118, 129
  reporting rape 116
  teenagers as victims 20, 23–24
National Domestic Violence Hotline
  43, 174
National Institute of Justice
  children and rape 78
  college rapes 27, 80
  drugs, alcohol, and rape 30
  ethnicity and rape 165
National Institute on Drug Abuse
  31, 80
National Juvenile Online
  Victimization study 66
National Runaway Switchboard
  67
National Violence Against Women
  Survey
  age of victims 78
  drugs, alcohol, and rape 80
  intimate partner violence 125
  rape rates 117–118
  reporting rape 26
National Women's Health
  Information Center 174
National Women's Study 120

NCAC (National Children's Advocacy
  Center) 174
nursing homes 138–139

O

Office of Juvenile Justice and
  Delinquency Prevention 136, 158
Office on Violence Against Women
  29
*Online Victimization of Youth: 5
  Years Later* (Wolak et al.) 65

P

Parrot, Andrea 55
pedophiles. *See* children and rape;
  children and sexual violence
A Perfect Cause 138
Pew Internet study 66–67
pornography 16, 152–153
post-traumatic stress disorder (PTSD)
  33, 109, 121, 126
predatory drugs 31, 39–40, 62,
  141–142
pregnancy 96, 114, 121
Prevent Child Abuse America 175
prevention, proactive **83–90**. *See
  also* safe areas, establishing
  children, strategies for 22
  community efforts 90
  date rape 32–33
  education 84, 89–90
  gang rape 56–57
  lowering risk 84–87
  predatory drugs 41
  self-defense 88–89
  sexual harassment 148–149
prevention, reactive **91–95**, 96. *See
  also* safe areas, establishing
Prison Rape Elimination Act 136,
  138
prisons 134–136
Protection of Children Against
  Exploitation Act 152

Protect Law 153

Psychology of Women Quarterly 79

PTSD. *See* post-traumatic stress
  disorder (PTSD) 33, 109, 121, 126

Q

questions and answers
  children and rape 60
  children and sexual violence
    151–152
  defining rape 41
  drugs, alcohol, and rape 125–126
  effects of rape 78–79
  emergency contraception 96
  evidence collection 112–113
  fighting an attacker 91
  gang rape 54
  Internet predators 70
  media and rape 105
  nursing homes and rape 138
  reporting rape 44
  school safety 131
  sexual harassment 144–145, 150
  statutory rape 72
  teenagers as victims 20
  victims of rape 29, 84, 164
  war, rape in 111

R

RAD (Rape Aggression Defense)
  88

Rape, Abuse, & Incest National
  Network (RAINN) 43, 62, 124, 166,
  175

*Rape, Sexual Violence and HIV in
  Conflict and Post-Conflict Zones*
  110

Rape Aggression Defense (RAD) 88

Rape and Sexual Assault (Koss) 30

*Rape and Sexual Assault: Reporting
  to Police and Medical Attention*
  (Rennison) 118

rape in war 108–111

rape kits and evidence collection
  111–116
  collecting evidence 111–113
  sexual assault nurse examiners
    (SANE) 114
  unprocessed kits 114–115

Rape: The Misunderstood Crime
  (Allison) 77

rape trauma syndrome 126. *See also*
  post-traumatic stress disorder (PTSD)

rapists. *See also* Internet predators;
  male role in rape
  characteristics of 28, 54
  of children 126–127
  psychological impairments of
    17–18
  social skills, lack of 16–17
  and statutory rape 158

religion 48–50, **96–98**

Rennison, Callie Marie 118

reporting rape
  Internet predators, reporting
    69–70
  and male victims 169–170
  reasons for not reporting 35–36,
    42
  relief after 161
  as response to rape 62
  statistics 1, 40, 166
  statutory rape 158–159
  and support for victims 59

Rickett, V. I. 27

Rohypnol (flunitrazepam) 31, 40,
  62, 142

Roman Catholic Church. *See* Catholic
  Church

S

safe areas, establishing **129–134**.
  See also prevention, reactive
  community safety 133–134
  home safety 129–130
  school safety 130–133

The Safer Society Foundation 175
Safe School Helpline 130, 175
Sanday, Peggy 76, 99
Sandhu, D. S. 146
SANE (sexual assault nurse examiners) 114–115
SAVE (Students Against Violence Everywhere) 132
self-defense 88–89
Senate Judiciary Committee 35
sex offender registry 103
Sex Offenses and Offenders 8
Sex Roles 78, 80, 149–150
Sex Rules 150
Sexual Abuse 169
sexual abuse in institutions **134–139**
  juvenile detention facilities 136–138
  mental institutions 134–135
  nursing homes 138–139
  prisons 135–136
sexual assault, types of **139–146**
  child abuse 144
  exhibitionism 144
  and rape 4–6, 139–142
  sexual harassment 145–146
  voyeurism 142–144
sexual assault nurse examiners (SANE) 114–115
Sexual Assault on Campus: The Problem and the Solution (Bohmer & Parrot) 55
sexual harassment 67, 145–146, **146–150**
Sexual Harassment: It's Not Academic 149
The Sexuality Information and Education Council of the United States 175–176
sexually transmitted diseases (STDs)
  medical examination for 62, 95
  in prisoners 135
  and SANE nurses 114

statistics 121
  as weapon of war 110–111
The Sexual Victimization of College Women 80
shield laws 73–74, 106
Smith, C. A. 17
society and rape **99–104**
  about 3–4
  blaming victims 103–104
  changing attitudes 170
  cultural expectations 77–80, 100–101
  International Women's Day 104
  marital rape 101–102
  Megan's Laws 103
  and public health 99–100
  rape script 102
  social influences 15–16
sodomy 142
statistics **116–123**
  children and rape 20, 22–23
  children and sexual violence 151–154
  date rape 26–27
  drugs, alcohol, and rape 37
  gender of victims and perpetrators 60, 75
  history of abuse 137
  male victims 168–169
  perpetrators 119–122
  rape rates 7, 85, 117–118, 124
  special populations 122–123
statutory rape **154–160**
  about 5, 23–24, 25, 141, 151
  and consent of minor 72
  and Internet predators 68
  laws about 155–158
  reporting requirements 158–159
  victims and offenders 158
Statutory Rape: A Guide to State Laws and Reporting Requirements 156, 157

STDs. *See* sexually transmitted diseases (STDs)
stigma of rape **160–165**
  court appearances 163–165
  legal impact 162–163
  psychological impact 160–161
  and underreporting 6–8
Students Against Violence Everywhere (SAVE) 132
support for victims. *See* help and support
Survivors of Incest Anonymous 176

T

Take Back the Night 50
Teens, Crime, and the Community (TCC) 133
teens speak
  alcohol and rape 38
  date rape 34
  fighting an attacker 92
  gang rape 55–56
  male role in rape 79–80
  prevention 89
  rape, defined 140
  reporting rape 45, 62–63
  school safety 132–133
  statutory rape 159–160
  stigma of rape 162
terminology 5–6
Thomas, Matt 88
Tyson, Mike 82

V

The Vagina Monologues 51
V-day 51

victims of rape, female **165–167**
victims of rape, male **168–171**
Violence Against Women 148
Violence Against Women, Identifying Risk Factors 151–152
Violence Against Women Act 101
Violence and Victims 167
voyeurism 142–144

W

Warshaw, Robin 54
WHO. *See* World Health Organization (WHO)
Wieman, C. M. 27
Wired Safety 70
Wolak, J. 65
Women's Equity in Access to Care and Treatment 110
Women's Health America 176
World Health Organization (WHO)
  genital mutilation 52
  marital rape 101
  rapists, male 75
  risk factors for sexual violence 76
  social factors in rape 99
  violence against women 104

X

Xanax (alprazolam) 31

Y

Youth Relationships Program 44–45
Youth Risk Behavior Surveillance System (YRBSS) 27, 117, 121, 176
Youth Safety Corps (YSC) 133